Reflections *on* Doctors

Reflections *on* Doctors

Nurses' Stories about Physicians and Surgeons

~

Terry Ratner, RN, MFA

EDITOR

KAPLAN PUBLISHING

This publication is designed to provide accurate and authoritative information in regard to the subject matter covered. It is sold with the understanding that the publisher is not engaged in rendering legal, accounting, or other professional service. If legal advice or other expert assistance is required, the services of a competent professional should be sought.

While the stories in *Reflections on Doctors* are based on real events, names, places, and other details have been changed for the sake of privacy.

© 2008 Kaplan, Inc.

Published by Kaplan Publishing, a division of Kaplan, Inc.
1 Liberty Plaza, 24th Floor
New York, NY 10006

Printed in the United States of America

Library of Congress Cataloging-in-Publication Data

Reflections on doctors : nurse's stories about physicians and surgeons / [edited by] Terry Ratner.
       p. ;   cm.
   ISBN 978-1-4277-9825-1
   1. Nurse and physician--Anecdotes. I. Ratner, Terry.
   [DNLM: 1. Physician-Nurse Relations--Personal Narratives.
   2. Nurses--Personal Narratives. 3. Physicians--Personal Narratives.
   WY 87 R332 2008]

   RT86.4.R45 2008
   610.73'0699--dc22

                                                                2008028267

2008
10 9 8 7 6 5 4 3 2 1
ISBN-13: 978-1-4277-9825-1

Kaplan Publishing books are available at special quantity discounts to use for sales promotions, employee premiums, or educational purposes. Please email our Special Sales Department to order or for more information at kaplanpublishing@kaplan.com, or write to Kaplan Publishing, 1 Liberty Plaza, 24th Floor, New York, NY 10006.

Contents

Introduction

"No man, not even a doctor, ever gives
any other definition of what a nurse
should be than this—'devoted and obedient.'
This definition would do just as well
for a porter. It might even do for a horse."

— Florence Nightingale, 1859

NURSING HAS BEEN called the oldest of arts and the youngest of professions. The number of nurses worldwide totals more than 11 million, yet this profession is still difficult to describe and continues to be poorly understood by nurses, physicians, and the public in general.

In 1859, Florence Nightingale wrote, "The elements of nursing are all but unknown." While this statement remains true in a sense even now, the roles and responsibilities of nurses and physicians have been refined considerably.

The nursing profession has evolved over time, and with it, the scope of a nurse's distinct responsibilities. The role of a nurse has long been defined in relation to physicians; they were bound at the hip, which limited nurses' scope of practice and autonomy. With different educational paths and scopes of practice, nurses and physicians now work side by side.

The word "doctor" stems from the earliest role doctors had with nurses—the role of teacher (the Latin meaning of doctor). Before 1929, a major portion of a nurse's teachings were done by doctors. In the 1940s nurses started to vocalize their feelings about nursing care and their need to distinguish themselves in the medical profession. They began to concentrate on the needs of a patient, a focus much different from the one of "handmaiden" to a physician.

Whether we call them doctors or physicians, whether we think of them as teachers or as healers, they are vital team players in today's healthcare industry. The relationship between the fraternity of doctors, once a rigid hierarchy that placed physicians firmly in charge, and the sorority of nurses has changed throughout the years.

Reflections on Doctors is an anthology about nurses and physicians inseparably intertwined in a variety of settings, yet distinctly different in their specific roles. The distinctions are clear—patient outcomes are dependent upon the physician's skills in diagnosing and the nurse's continuous observations and their ability to communicate the right information to the appropriate care provider.

The nurses who have contributed to this important anthology represent a spectrum of voices and perspectives. Nurses, some doctors themselves by virtue of a PhD, reflect upon their work alongside physicians. Some have been in nursing for decades, while others are newer to the field. Some have had only positive working relationships, while others have experienced some bumps along the way. The majority of these nurses have witnessed considerable changes in the nurse-physician relationship over time. They are our messengers, our heroes, and our scribes.

Their voices are frustrated at times, often controversial, but seldom sentimental. The sharing of their stories contributes to the revolutionary change in our image of nurses; instead of responding to authority with unquestioning obedience, nurses are trained to question, seek answers, and to express themselves verbally.

This diverse collection of essays, written in remarkable prose, contains intimate nursing notes, not found in textbooks or in a patient's chart. Nurses reveal their experiences with honesty, compassion, and a genuine concern for their profession. They cover a

variety of themes, from the role of nurses and physicians to the scope of their respective practice.

Keith Carlson and Angela Posey-Arnold write
about strong leadership and how it impacts a health
organization. Karen Klein dares to write about the
consequences of deferring to a doctor's authority and
standing up for what she believes in. You'll find nurses
like Heidi Lipka and Carolyn Lounsbury who use
humor as an antidote for headstrong doctors. Pamela
Gonzalez's "Smart Enough Not to Be a Doctor" por-
trays public perceptions of nurses and doctors, while
Nancy Leigh Harless writes about the misconceptions
nurses have about doctors. Defined roles for physicians and nurses are addressed by Anna Gregory's and
Cara Muhlhahn's fine essays.

In these pages, nurses reveal themselves as fully
human as they talk about their personal relationships
with doctors, the doctor-patient relationship, and the
importance of feeling comfortable with patients' emotional needs. One provocative essay follows a patient's
descent into the world of illness—a story, according
to Cortney Davis, caregivers rarely hear. You'll find
nurses like Adrienne Zurub writing about the dynamics of gender, "the encompassing fog of testosterone,"
and how it affects the bond between nurses and doctors. The stories in this anthology bring readers behind

closed doors, into the OR, to the bedside, and to the *ambulantas* in the fields of Kosovo.

A reader's guide, providing opportunities for further discussion of these provocative stories, is located in the back of the book. This is an ideal way for readers to hold a "meeting of the minds" and begin crucial conversations in hopes of increasing their understanding of the nurse-physician relationship.

Whether you're a new grad, seasoned nurse, or someone interested in understanding the dynamics of communication between physicians and nurses, you'll have a front row seat under the big top of our healthcare arena—a view of the past and present, and a glimpse of the future. Welcome to our world, *Reflections on Doctors: Nurses' Stories about Physicians and Surgeons*. We hope it pleases, shocks, surprises, and astounds you.

Reflections *on* Doctors

Refusing
Doctors' Orders

~

Karen Klein, RN

In my 24 years as a nurse I have refused doctors' orders on only two occasions. Refusal to carry out a doctor's order is the right of every nurse who feels the order is not appropriate. Doctors always have the right to carry the order out themselves, if they so choose, while the nurse should chart the refusal and the reason.

The first occasion was when I worked in a small, six-bed surgical step-down unit for patients who were too well for intensive care (ICU), but needed more monitoring than could be provided on a general surgical unit. It was a two-room unit—male and female—with three beds per room, connected by a short, narrow hallway. One nurse was assigned to each room. The nurses' desk was literally in the same small room with the patients.

I worked the 8 PM–8 AM shift. One night I had a male patient who had just had a triple bypass the day prior but had done so well that he was moved to our unit. All night I noted he slept well. In "hospital speak" this means he got four solid hours of sleep. At one point he had removed his oxygen nasal cannula for comfort, so I was sure to monitor his oxygen levels via a pulse oximeter, which I had previously applied like a Band-Aid to one fingernail. His oxygen levels remained stable. He was in no distress. In the morning, I assisted him out of bed and he did his ablutions with minimal assistance, never requiring oxygen nor becoming short of breath. He did his post-heart surgery spirometer exercises with no problem.

Just after he finished, while still sitting in the chair, the chief surgical resident and his team visited the patient while they were on their morning rounds. The chief was concerned about the patient's chest X-ray, which showed a possible atelectasis (small collapses) in the left lower lung. When we were out of the patient's earshot, I questioned the finding. Rather than acknowledge my concerns, the doctor demanded, in front of the entire team, that I nasally suction the patient. He made a point of telling one intern to be sure to write on the order sheet that the patient was to be suctioned every hour.

I was still a fairly new nurse with only three years of experience, but I summoned the courage and verbally refused to carry out that order. I just couldn't imagine going up to that man and shoving a long tube down his nose trying to get it down a lung to suck out…what? The man could cough up whatever he needed to clear his own lungs. I had literally sat at a desk behind his bed the entire night listening to his breathing and that patient had no atelectasis. I didn't care what the chest X-ray showed. Besides, the suctioning process itself is distressing as it takes away the patient's airway and is monumentally uncomfortable for an alert person. It can even cause heartbeat irregularities (cardiac disrhythmias). I told the doctor all of this. I could see cautious looks on the interns' faces as they looked at me, then the doctor, then back at me. This chief resident, who was well known to be a bit arrogant, was on the spot. He was indignant, insisting that one of the interns return in an hour to suction the patient. Then he stormed off with his lackeys in tow.

An hour later, much to my surprise, I was visited not by one of the interns, but by the chief resident. More surprisingly, he had come to cancel the suctioning order, telling me that he had fully reviewed the patient's medical history and saw that the patient had an old war wound, which had damaged his left lower lung, so it had only appeared as an atelectasis on the X-ray. Most surprising of all, he apologized. I responded, "Look, we're on the same side. We both want what's best for the patient. So just always remember—listen to the nurses!"

He admitted that this incident had taught him the value of the nurses' input regarding patient assessment, treatment, and care. He said that in the future he would be sure to take the nurses' input into serious consideration before determining a patient's treatment course. He confessed that although he knew he came off as arrogant at times, it was really just insecurity. He really just wanted to be a great surgeon. I smiled and said, "If you continue to show the integrity, humility, and openness to learning that you just demonstrated, I have no doubt you will be."

THE OTHER OCCASION I refused a doctor's order did not turn out quite so well. I was working in an urban emergency room. A patient was brought in with a stab wound in his right upper abdomen. He arrived by emergency medical services on a stretcher, lying flat and not wearing any oxygen, with no visible sign of respiratory distress. He was fully conscious and speaking his native language—Korean. For some reason, though, the ER attending physician called for a setup for the insertion of a chest tube. This is done when the lung collapses, in order to reinflate it. But the patient had no obvious signs of lung collapse. The trauma team had been called but not yet arrived, so it was myself, an ER resident, this attending, and the medics in the trauma room with the patient.

I began to work on the patient, placing him on oxygen, inserting IVs, and attaching him to monitoring devices, but I held off on the chest tube setup. It was pretty clear that the patient was not in need of one but since anything is technically possible with a right upper quadrant stab wound, I called for a stat portable chest X-ray. The doctor, however, did not want to wait the five minutes for the X-ray to be taken and developed. He insisted again that I set up for a chest tube. The insertion is quite painful, as anyone who has ever had one inserted while conscious can tell you. Basically the doctor sticks a small spear into the patient's side between the ribs. The "spear" (trocar) has a catheter over it, which gets left in when the spear is removed. Then that catheter (tube) is hooked up to a device to maintain positive pressure. It almost instantly fully reinflates a lung but then the person's act of breathing assists in complete reinflation slowly over time—days—as the lung heals itself from whatever injury made it collapse.

I told the attending that I didn't think the patient needed a chest tube and that we should wait for the X-ray. He told me he didn't care what I thought and again insisted I do the setup. I got the tray but dawdled in the setup long enough for the X-ray to be taken. In anger the doctor came up behind me and patted my back twice, saying, "Come on, move it," meaning, hurry up with the setup. As he walked to my side, I noticed his gloves had blood all over them. I strongly suspected there was now blood on the back of my lab coat, soaking through my uniform.

"If you want to insist on putting in the chest tube, you can do the setup. I'm refusing the order," I told him and I walked out of the room. I immediately asked the nurse I was working with that day to care for the patient since he was a trauma victim and needed a nurse.

As I turned away, headed for the nurses' lounge, she remarked, "Oh my God, you have blood all over the back of your lab coat!" I just kept walking. When I got into the lounge, I carefully removed the coat. Sure enough, as I had suspected, there were two bloody handprints on my back. I was incensed.

I saved the white coat with the bloody handprints in a bag and the following day showed it to my nurse manager. I wanted to report not only his dangerous, erratic behavior toward me, but his poor medical judgment as well—demonstrated by his demanding a chest tube for a patient who clearly did not need one—proven five minutes later by the chest X-ray results. My nurse manager took the bloody lab coat and said she'd get back to me.

The next day, she called me into her office. I was really floored when she told me to buy myself another lab coat that the hospital would reimburse me for, adding that they prefer I not discuss the incident with anyone. She said they wanted the incident to go away quietly. I questioned her about the doctor's erratic behavior and the possible harm he might one day cause a patient but she held her ground. Inside, I was livid. But I responded, "Thanks for the new lab coat," and left the office. I later went and bought the most expensive lab coat I could find. But unfortunately for the nurse manager I was unable to abide by her other request.

The nurse who had seen the bloody jacket that day had already told many of the nurses about the incident. In hospitals, word spreads fast and lingers long. In fact, one person compared me to Monica Lewinsky because I saved the jacket as evidence. For a long while after, I would be teasingly referred to as Monica by some of the nurses.

As for the doctor, he left that ER shortly after the incident. I don't really know whatever became of him. Hopefully, he got the help he needed.

Please Help
My Son Not Die

~

Nancy Leigh Harless, NP

*There is no mistaking love. You feel it in
your heart. It is the common fiber of life,
the flame that lights our soul, energizes
our spirit and supplies passion to our lives.
It is our connection to God and to each other.*

— Elizabeth Kubler-Ross

MY FIRST DAY in the field in Kosovo was June 6, 2000. I had been in the country for two weeks. My luggage, lost in transit, arrived the day before. I saw it as a good sign.

However, over the next three months I found myself spiraling down into the abyss we call evil. I saw and heard of things I had never even imagined.

Thankfully, I was also uplifted to extraordinary heights when I witnessed the kindness, compassion, and love that mark the other end of the continuum of human behavior.

The medical project was part of a larger international humanitarian mission to implement modern healthcare in the Balkans as part of the war recovery effort. As a nurse practitioner specializing in women's healthcare, my job was to train Kosovar doctors and nurses to provide excellent prenatal care. And because the notion of consulting a healthcare provider throughout pregnancy was foreign to the village women, we had to sell the idea through community education and one-on-one interactions.

At first, I felt uncomfortable with the idea that I, a nurse practitioner from the States, was to teach Kosovar doctors. However, once the history was explained, it made perfect sense. Medical training for the Albanian Kosovar doctors had been thwarted by the political unrest over the years, and they were forced to develop a separate, parallel system of medical education from their Serbian counterparts.

Their training was lacking in many ways. A nurse's training consisted of a high school diploma. Doctors attended the same high school followed by only four years of training. My job was to help fill in the gaps of their knowledge base and provide guidance through didactic studies in the office and on-the-job supervised experience in the *ambulantas*, small, sparsely furnished clinics scattered around the countryside. We began as a team of five women. From Kosovo, there were two doctors, Linda and Mirvete, and two nurses, Bedreji and Dejetare. And then there was me. We loaded the van with all the supplies needed to take to the village of Sllatina. There we would hold a clinic for women, providing education, exams, and medications. We would refer serious problems to the nearest health house, the equivalent to a small hospital, and offer transportation if needed. We provided community education to the people who clustered about the *ambulanta* to see what was happening. Education would be the most important thing we would bring to the villages.

In Kosovo, women and babies balanced precariously on the brink between life and death. Kosovo is part of Europe, but not the modern Europe of travel posters. Healthcare in Kosovo, particularly in the villages, operated like it did several hundred years ago. Women weren't seen by a healthcare provider throughout their pregnancies, nor were they educated in the warning signs of a problem in the pregnancy—signs that indicate the mother's or her baby's life might be in danger. Because many of the villagers couldn't read or write, we prepared booklets with pictures depicting the dangers. They showed bleeding, swelling of feet or face, headache and blurry vision, lack of fetal movement, gush of water, persistent backache, or contractions before 37 weeks. The booklets reinforced what we taught.

Neonatal tetanus, virtually an unknown problem in the developed world, was a common cause of newborn death in Kosovo. By simply providing the mother with two doses of vaccine during her pregnancy, that problem could be eliminated.

We packed the van with everything we needed to hold a clinic. One large trunk contained medicines and vitamins, another housed basic medical equipment and supplies: blood pressure cuffs, stethoscopes, and weight scales for both mothers and babies. Five-gallon jerricans held the water needed for hand washing.

The *ambulantas* were rough, small buildings. Some had electricity or running water. They had three small rooms. We used one for a waiting room; the other two served as exam rooms. If there was a bathroom, it was the size of a small closet with a hole in the floor for squatting purposes.

Just as we finished loading the van, an old woman arrived, dressed in a simple, navy-blue cotton dress and sensible shoes. She had a large port-wine birthmark that covered the left side of her face and the right side of her mouth drooped, causing spittle to collect in the corner when she talked. I suspected that she had experienced a stroke sometime in the past. I estimated that she was in her mid-sixties but learned later that she was much younger. Hard times and horror had taken their toll, turned her hair gray, and left deep creases of worry on her already disfigured face. But when I looked into her eyes, I saw only kindness and the twinkle of humor that I would later learn was the hallmark of Dr. Drita, one of the doctors who was to join our team.

The old woman spoke to Dr. Linda in Albanian. From Linda's expression, it seemed she delivered an upsetting message.

"What is it?" I asked.

"She is Dr. Drita. She says she is part of us. She says she is to work with our team. But she is a pediatrician. We are women's care. I think it is a mistake," Linda said.

Puzzled, I extended my hand to the old woman and introduced myself. "Hello, I'm Nancy."

"*Une' jam* Drita," she responded with a warm smile, eyes crinkling at the corners.

I excused myself from the group and went inside the office to try to call the main office to determine if, indeed, Dr. Drita was part of my staff.

This morning the telephone in the office was dead, which was not unusual, as communications in

Kosovo were often a challenge. It was unusual, however, that the shortwave radio wasn't able to squeak out a brief static-filled message to headquarters.

Frustrated, I found the office manager, Laura, and asked, "Do you know if a Dr. Drita is supposed to be with my team today?"

"The pediatrician? She finally showed up? Yeah, Rose has been expecting her for a month," Laura said.

Only one week ago I had taken over the team from Rose, a petite redheaded German doctor who had been in Kosovo since the war began. She had worked with this group for the past six months. The staff had one week to adapt to me as their new leader, and they were still adjusting to losing their beloved Rose. Now I asked them to accept another new doctor as well. Like people everywhere adjusting to change, they resisted the idea at first.

Packed like sardines, the doctors, nurses, a driver, and I squeezed into the van filled with supplies. The tension in the tight van was palpable as we drove down the bumpy road to the village.

When we arrived at the *ambulanta* — a tiny, stark clinic without running water, Dr. Drita wandered off to find the bathroom. As we unpacked the van, the other four attacked me and prattled like children. "It isn't fair!" complained Nurse Bedreji.

"We are too many," spat Dr. Mirvete.

"We are only women's care. Why do we need a pediatrician?" questioned Nurse Dejetare.

"We are already too crowded," whined Dr. Linda.

On and on and on it went, and this was only the part I understood. All four of the women spoke English. Dr. Linda and Nurse Bedreji continued to berate me in English. Frustrated, Dr. Mirvete and Nurse Dejetare shifted into Albanian. They were relentless!

I did the best I could to explain and apologize for not preparing them for the sudden change and then told them firmly I expected them all to help make Dr. Drita feel part of the team.

"Remember, we are MCH—*maternal child health*," I reminded them. "Dr. Drita is here to help us with the child part of our job."

All conversation in the room suddenly shifted to Albanian. I think that one of them may have even called me a name, but I could only imagine what they were saying. Inwardly, I groaned. *Only one week in the country and already I'm the enemy. This is not a good beginning.*

I didn't understand why they opposed the new doctor. Perhaps simply it was too many changes to accept. And they were accustomed to Rose. They didn't know yet if they could trust me. There is safety in a routine and comfort in the status quo.

Because they had lived through a war, each of these women carried a long personal history that was more than enough reason to understand their insecurity and resistance to change. Luckily, it was not a busy clinic that morning, and only one woman was waiting for us when we arrived. She was a thin woman with no upper teeth and only three lower. She was wearing a dirty white T-shirt, two sizes too large, and baggy black pants. She brought her five-day-old son swaddled in a cloth, like a little pig-in-a-blanket sausage. He was her third son. Her first two babies lived only one month. She was certain they died of hunger.

"My baby is so big. My breast is so small," she said, hanging her head.

She asked for help to buy milk from a can for her baby, but we had no assistance of that kind, and, in fact—for myriad reasons—encouraged breast-feeding for all of our patients. The antibodies that pass through to a baby in mother's milk alone are reason enough to encourage breast-feeding. Breast milk is also the perfect combination of nutrients for optimal infant health and growth. There is some thought that nursing helps with mother-baby bonding and decreases blood loss after delivery. It also helps the uterus return to its original size and tone, and it facilitates losing excess weight after delivery. It's free and it comes already warmed in a clean container with no need to sterilize bottles or boil water.

Dr. Linda did the woman's postpartum assessment and found the woman was recovering well and was healthy. Her only concerns were for her baby. Both Dr. Linda and Dr. Mirvete tried to reassure her and tell her about all the advantages of breast-feeding.

They looked to me for guidance. I showed her baby positioning and encouraged nutrition and fluids. With the doctors translating, I assured the woman that her breast would produce all the milk that her baby needed, but I could tell by the nervous, tight twitch of her body and the pinched expression in her eyes she was not satisfied.

"Please help my son not die," she pleaded.

I felt a knot in the pit of my stomach as Nurse Dejetare translated her plea to me. Swallowing, I suggested it might help if Dr. Drita, the unwelcome pediatrician, examined the baby boy.

"Yes, the pediatrician!" said Dr. Linda, and then hurried off to find Dr. Drita.

It had to be providence that brought this particular patient with her special concerns to the clinic that morning because what I witnessed over the next hour was nothing short of a miracle. Unlike the younger members on the medical team, Dr. Drita had not trained in the back-alley educational system of medical schools held in basements and garages. She received her training prior to the unrest in her country, when institutions were intact. Dr. Drita was not just an adequate doctor; she was an outstanding one. With more than 20 years of experience and a passion and talent for teaching, she proceeded to perform the most thorough newborn baby exam I have ever witnessed—anywhere.

Speaking in a low, calm voice, Dr. Drita slowly unwrapped the baby boy from his swaddling. Beginning at his head she gently palpated his fontanel, the soft spot on top on his head, and explained to the mother it should be soft but not sunken.

"This is one way you will know your baby is drinking enough," she told the young mother. "If his soft spot was depressed, it would tell us he was dehydrated, but see how nice and soft your baby's head is? Perfect!" Dr. Drita praised.

She gently palpated the baby's abdomen and pointed out there was no discharge, no redness, no swelling around his umbilicus—his belly button. "There should be no redness. No discharge. See how perfect this baby's tummy is? Perfect!" Dr. Drita said, pointing to his tiny tummy.

As she continued to examine him, she explained every step to the mother and to the staff. She performed a neurological exam and demonstrated the doll's eyes reflex, a phenomenon that causes a baby's eyes to open when gently pulled from prone to sitting position.

Using another phenomenon called the "walking reflex," she showed how he could "walk" when held in a standing position with his feet touching the table. As he lifted his legs in a stepping movement, Drita reassured the mother. "See, your baby is strong and well."

Drita was not only an amazing doctor, but also a spiritual healer. As she demonstrated respect, patience, and kindness, the mother's ability to believe in herself blossomed. The staff stood by engrossed as they learned how to properly evaluate a newborn. At the same time—and even more importantly—they saw the young mother's confidence grow before their very eyes. Her shoulders eased. The tight, pinched look around her eyes relaxed into a little smile.

When Dr. Drita finished with the exam, she reswaddled the baby, placed him in his mother's arms, and instructed her how to feed him. When the mother complied, Dr. Drita applauded. "Bravo! You see, your body will provide for your son."

It was a light-filled moment. All the doctors and nurses began to clap. The mother was smiling from ear to ear, a wide but toothless grin, and repeating, *"Faleminderit, faleminderit"* ("thank you, thank you") over and over again. Having Dr. Drita on the team was no longer a problem.

Miracles happen. They happen whenever, wherever there is great love. Bravo, Dr. Drita. Bravo!

A Truth about Cats and Dogs

~

Adrienne Zurub, RN, MA, CNOR

Mornings are not supposed to smell like burning flesh with wispy twirls of flesh smoke moving sensually and methodically toward the cluster of operating-room lights. Morning sounds should not be muffled weeping or verbalized grimaces. The sounds of morning should not allow the normalcy of the electric saw making its way through the guardian bone of sternum, thus literally exposing someone's heart to the world. Yet for me these were my mornings for more than 25 years.

This setting, barbaric in any sense of the word, was the backdrop of my experience as a cardiothoracic

surgical RN (formerly) on the open heart-heart transplant team at Cleveland Clinic. These ORs were my
battleground and playground. Those experiences and
visuals, and their accompanying sensations—good and
bad—became the foreground of my holistic collage.

The fugitive truth is that those sounds, that
weeping and those grimaces by patients (and staff
alike) become talismans that we (nurses and surgeons)
carry the rest of our respective lives. Often, I viewed
the surgeons I worked with as automatons in the OR.
And indeed some surgeons acquire this "distancing"
veneer in order to do the necessary work.

In our cardiothoracic operating rooms, an over-
arching competitive environment exists. Arrogance,
entitlement, outstanding talents (nurses and surgeons),
and palpable confidence dominate the entire operating-
room suites. A nurse pushes herself or himself through
this encompassing fog of testosterone. I say *testosterone*
because the surgeons, the ones who are in charge, are
all male. To work in this environment, one has to have
the personality and the chutzpah—the balls—to think
quickly and react perfectly. Weakness or hesitation is
normally not considered an option.

So it was with great surprise that I was approached
one late evening, as I sat at the cardiac control desk,
by a new staff surgeon who had lost a patient. During
the exchange, I came to realize how remarkable the

distancing has to be in order for this new staff guy to do his job and perform extraordinary feats of surgery. I also realized in those moments that I was the one who resided in a protective callus acquired from years of experience, years of death, and the pain of knowing. My sense of efficacy allowed that this OR death and its cognitive talisman would be one of many that he (like me) will carry the rest of our lives in our efforts to help others.

In this one illuminating moment, the distance and power dynamic between the two forces, that of nurse and doctor, are somehow bridged. Here we are one. The hospital-induced power differential is turned on its head, as I, being the experienced nurse, am deemed the wise one, the resource, and a confidante. There was simply in our communication the active current of humanness that permeated the space between us.

He stood before me, crushed and battered at his first operating-room death. He wept openly before me, making me uncomfortable. I am accustomed to fits of rage, screaming, yelling, sulkiness, and a bit of (okay, a lot of) berating for the failure, the mistake, and falling short of expectations and the realization that they (heart surgeons) too are simply human.

He may realize that no matter what surgical algorithm he performs on patients that present to him, some patients will rightfully die. This is not an indictment, or an acquiescence of hope, but simply the reality of man versus destiny or a divine force.

This OR beckons to those patients who have no place else to go. Those who have been told by the second and third opinion to "go home and comfortably die." We are the last hope for these extremely high-acuity patients... and sometimes their last stop. Although many of the patients know this upon entering our OR, their families do not always understand.

Years ago, the surgeons appeared to love the thrill of the cases that were deemed impossible and time-consuming. Those guys were machinelike, churning out successes and making history. The newer guys are more... human. They desire success, but not at the expense of their family and a life.

So, I am heartened by this surgeon's 21st-century attitude. It is an attitude that, at least for now, shows that he does not need to step on me or my fellow colleagues. He is young and not yet institutionalized to the vagaries of our power hierarchy. Now he is willing to show his vulnerability.

I wonder what this new surgeon's—the one with the size-eight hands—reaction will be in, say, ten years or even a year from now. I wonder if this loss will be his "Moby Dick" in the continual pursuit and war against heart disease. Which patients will stay with him and further hone his skills with their respective challenges? Which patients will leave the remnants of themselves forever on his psyche...as they have left the talismans of themselves on me? Right now, he and I are partners.

Every Patient Tells a Story

~

Cheryl Dellasega, PhD

WE ARE CREATURES of words: beautiful words, idle words, hurtful words, empty words, and sometimes, healing words. We have words for who we are and what we do, words for where we work and live, and even words for the ways in which we relate to each other.

The words of medicine are often secret words, laden with meaning that escapes the untrained: agonal breathing, glomerular nephritis, metastasized cancer, retrograde ejaculation. It's easy to get lost in the poetry of medical words, using them to tell patients stories about the most significant aspects of their lives, and then considering our job done.

Yet to truly share words requires both a speaker and a listener. In day-to-day dealing with people, it's all too easy to depend on the first and forget about the latter. We don't hear the middle-aged man with Type 2 Diabetes Mellitus talk about his twin teenaged daughters' first prom the week before. An elderly widow's recollection of her prize in a ballroom dancing contest passes us by as we document our findings in her chart. A young woman's tale of pending divorce is overlooked in the search for the cause of her enlarged thyroid.

In the health professions, it happens every day. Lying in bed one night, I remember a moment right before lunch when a young woman began to tell me a story that was important to her. We were interrupted by the words of someone else, and although I told her I would listen to it later, I never did. The lost opportunity, signaled by the earnest look on her face, stayed with me for weeks.

The tendency to value our own words over those of patients was never more apparent to me than at a recent communication workshop for healthcare professionals. Along with dozens of other nurses, physicians, and therapists, I engaged in exercises designed to enhance our skills, yet the emphasis seemed to be all about speaking—and so little about listening. "Hearing" another person's story came to mean quickly responding to the spoken word through the lens of our own perception.

In the Quaker tradition, listening is deeper than receiving words. Discernment, or the receiving, sorting out, and understanding of a message, is at the heart of communication. Only through discernment can we truly "hear" the meaning of our patients' stories, and in receiving that message, we preserve the person in the patient.

RM was an 80-year-old man who fell at home and was brought to the emergency department (ED) by ambulance. On arrival, he was comatose and in respiratory distress; by the time an MRI revealed a massive subdural bleed he had already been intubated. Two of RM's sons and his wife had accompanied him to the ED. A resident and the ED doctor offered a medical story: neurosurgery could relieve intracranial pressure, but was unlikely to return him to baseline. There was a high probability of residual deficits.

RM's family opted against the surgery, so he was transferred to the intensive care unit (ICU), pending the arrival of his third son. Last rites were administered, but the family was adamant that RM be kept "alive." For the next twenty-four hours, a ventilator and a cocktail of medications kept his lungs breathing, heart beating, and kidneys functioning. As in the ED, he was not responsive to any external stimuli.

The morning of Day Two in the ICU, both physicians and nurses told RM's family more medical stories: destabilizing tendencies, Glasgow Scale score, accumulating complications. Dr. J, a palliative care physician, was consulted. He arrived in the room and offered to tell yet another medical story.

The family declined to hear it. After some moments of silence, Dr. J began to ask about RM: What was his job? Where had he lived? How many children did he have, and what did they do? Slowly, the story of RM emerged, as Dr. J listened. After they finished sharing their memories of RM, they were ready to hear what Dr. J had to say.

Gently, he interpreted the medical stories they'd already been told, tying the MRI results to the fall, describing how RM's past medical history influenced his current condition, and, finally, explaining the prognosis in light of RM's advance directive. When Dr. J stopped speaking, the family turned to each other with a shared understanding. They asked that the ventilator be discontinued in a few hours. At 4 PM, RM died as a father, husband, and human being instead of as "the subdural bleed in Room 8."

As healers, we are, in essence, tellers and receivers of stories. Not only did Dr. J spend more time with RM and his family than any other physician, he also saved the hospital thousands of dollars because of the events which took place after he listened to the story of RM. His greater gift was discerning what a grieving family really needed in order to begin coping with the life that had left them.

Home Delivery

~

Cara Muhlhahn, CNM

I LOVE MY WORK, love every one of my patients, love being in private practice. I derive incredible satisfaction as a home-birth midwife from helping women become mothers in the most natural, safe, and empowered way. But there are many uphill battles in this field, especially these days, when home-birth midwives still need to fight for legitimacy. Things are gradually changing for the better, but there are still so many misperceptions about who we are and what we do.

A compliment I received from one father says it all. He was fine with the idea of home birth from the beginning. But the baby came out not breathing and I had to do a neonatal resuscitation. It was the Fourth of

July. The dad had called 911, at my request, just in case the resuscitation was not a success—which it was. At the end, when I was cleaning up the birthing pool, he came up to me and complimented me on how well I'd done, and on my "professional comportment."

He was incredibly relieved that I could successfully perform a resuscitation when needed. I don't think he ever considered that it might be possible. At the time I thought, "What did he expect?" But in hindsight I understand that patients and their partners don't necessarily understand that we're medically trained birthing professionals.

Before meeting me, this new dad had probably expected me to be some touchy-feely, matronly hippie equipped to offer little more than moral support, a hand to hold, and maybe some arcane, esoteric "wisewoman's" wisdom—all of which is probably quite helpful. He didn't expect me to be the serious, capable clinician that I am. I'm sure that his image of a midwife was forever changed.

It's not just the general public who's confused, but doctors as well. And the fact that there are so many routes of entry into midwifery creates even more confusion within the field. There are CNMs (certified nurse midwives), like me; CMs (certified midwives); and CPMs (certified professional midwives). The various groups of midwives have different levels of education and are standardized and regulated by different bodies that often disagree about things like protocols for licensure. And then there are midwives who have come to the profession through an unregulated apprenticeship. This confusion makes it more difficult to win political gains and the trust of the women who are thinking about choosing midwives.

Among the most frustrating of our hurdles is American doctors' misconceptions, because the medical field and its governing bodies—the American College of Obstetrics and Gynecology (ACOG), for example—have such influence over public opinion. In February 2008, ACOG released a statement reiterating their opposition to home birth—rather ignorantly, especially when considering that 70 percent of births in Europe and Japan are done at home.

DESPITE THE MISCONCEPTIONS, there are still physicians who manage to support women making empowering choices. Some doctors have taken the time to understand what home birth is about and what midwives do, and they are very supportive of us and our patients. I have been fortunate to find some with whom I can work, and I am grateful for them and all their referrals to my practice. I work regularly with a perinatologist, a cardiologist, a hematologist, holistic gynecologist, assorted ob-gyns, pediatricians, and psychologists. When we work in tandem, supporting one another, great things can happen.

And hospitals aren't all bad. We couldn't do without them in cases of emergency. They have intelligent doctors, machines, high-tech equipment, and medications on hand that are great to have access to when things are abnormal or dangerous. They're just not great places for normal birth.

Here's an example of a great collaboration between a couple of doctors and a midwife, and ways in which a hospital can even be helpful in supporting home birth. Sabine, a German-born patient of mine, had her first baby with Dr. Jacques Moritz, an ob-gyn colleague. Everything went fine. Dr. Moritz sent her my way when he knew that she was seeking a home birth for her second child.

Sabine's second pregnancy went beautifully. The baby grew normally in the third trimester. At the 32-week point, the head should begin to present, and the doctor or midwife checks to see that it's doing so. Sabine's baby's head was in a position that we call *oblique*, which means that instead of being directly in the pelvis, right over the pubic bone, it was a bit off to the side.

Toward the end of a woman's pregnancy, the prenatal visits get closer. Each time I came to see Sabine, I saw that her baby's head was moving slowly from oblique to transverse. At each visit I gently coaxed it back into the center, without duress, checking in on the baby's heartbeat to see if it minded, and it didn't.

From about the 37th week of a woman's pregnancy until delivery, I see her even more frequently—about once a week. During that time with Sabine, I noticed that the baby's head was moving slowly up toward the fundus, the top of the uterus. It seemed the baby was sneaking into a breech presentation. This was especially interesting to me because it recalled what my mother had told me about my time in utero: how the doctor kept turning me, but by the time we'd return for the next visit, I would revert to breech position.

I knew there had to be a reason this baby was turning the way it was. So I decided to take Sabine in for a sonogram to see where the cord was. I had a sneaking suspicion that the cord was around the neck, which is not usually a problem and occurs in 40 percent of normal deliveries. In this case, however, I thought it might be responsible for the baby's continuous journey northward.

Sabine and I went together to my perinatologist, Dr. Franz Margono at Saint Vincent's Hospital. We notified her husband, Ronnie, about what was going on and he went to meet us there. Dr. Margono did the sonogram and determined that the cord was twice around the neck and gave us advice to not "*schwinger*" the baby, using the German word for "swing," although it sounded more like *schvingeh*.

We explored the underlying meaning of Dr. Margono's advice for the next two hours or so at dinner nearby, where Ronnie joined us. I explained the situation to them, and laid out all the options. The implication of what Dr. Margono said was that I shouldn't force the baby back into a vertex presentation. *Ay, ay, ay,* I thought. If we couldn't get the baby back into a vertex presentation, then our options were quickly narrowing to a cesarean section, at least as our perinatologist saw it. I had a feeling, though, that things weren't so bleak. My instincts told me there was a way for Sabine to fulfill her dream of a home birth—or at the very least a vaginal birth rather than a C-section.

So I came up with a plan. Up until our last visit, I had been gently urging the baby from oblique and transverse to vertex without a problem as evidenced by my Doppler fetal heart rate. Of course, I was wrestling with the part of me that saw fit to bring Sabine in for a sonogram in the first place because the head was continuously rising in her uterus. I phoned Dr. Moritz, Sabine's former obstetrician, and asked him if he could turn the baby in the hospital as a way of ensuring that the baby tolerated the turning. There we would be able to monitor the baby after the turning. This might mean that Sabine would be induced to get her labor started before the baby could turn back around. Then, we'd head back to their place for a home birth.

For her part, Sabine would have been happy if I had just turned her baby once more. But I felt cautious with this new information about the cord wrapped twice around the baby's neck, and felt the heat of Dr. Margono's wagging "*no schvingeh*" finger. At this point, I was reluctant to turn the baby. My gut was telling me not to and I felt compelled to listen to it. I was still optimistic about the chances for a home birth, although Ronnie finally confessed to Sabine that "I was happy to go along with the home birth as long as things remained low-risk, but things have changed."

Dr. Moritz agreed to my plan. But the day Sabine went in ended up being extremely busy at the hospital, an inadvertent blessing in disguise. Sabine and Ronnie were there all day. After a long wait, the baby was easily turned. The doctor who did the turning said that it was possible that the cord was actually just laying over the shoulder, not wrapped around the neck twice as it had appeared to Dr. Margono. He explained that sonography is not a perfect science.

Many hours after turning, the baby was monitored and doing fine. Dr. Moritz was supposed to stop by, but his office hours were keeping him. In the meantime, Ronnie called me to say that the doctor who turned the baby was pushing for a hospital delivery.

The doctor told him, "Hey, you've played with this baby enough. Let's just get him out." This made Ronnie really anxious. He didn't want to do anything that would put the baby at risk.

I asked Ronnie if he—a professor—thought that the doctor had presented him with a well-thought-out risk-benefit analysis of the situation that made sense to him, as I had done the other night at dinner.

"No," he allowed. But he was uncertain how to proceed—due, of course, to the weight the doctor's statement carried.

I said to Ronnie, "Maybe this doctor is just opposed to home birth." When pressed by Ronnie, he revealed his bias against it.

Sabine had no problem sticking to her guns in the face of all of these medical assessments. Ronnie was doing his best to conquer his own fears, which were being exploited by the doctor who'd turned the baby. I finally got Dr. Moritz on the phone while they were at the hospital, and we talked. He said the baby had been monitored there all day and was doing fine.

I asked him, "If Sabine and Ronnie want to go ahead with the home birth, would you take us back in the hospital in the event that the baby experienced any distress?" The reason this had to be negotiated at that point was because I didn't feel comfortable, in the event of transfer, bringing Sabine back to Saint Vincent's having *schvinged*, albeit in the hospital under surveillance for the whole day.

Dr. Moritz said, "Sure." My kind of doctor.

Ronnie and Sabine came across town to my office. We made a plan for induction that night so the baby wouldn't have a chance to turn back around. The induction plan involved administration of castor oil. I decided to sleep at their house, Doppler-armed so as to make everyone—including myself—comfortable with the baby's status.

I listened to the baby all night. The signs were all good. The castor oil kicked in gradually and the labor proceeded slowly during the course of the day, as some second labors do. Sabine's doula was there. Things just didn't seem to be moving and so we all made a plan to go take a walk on the roof of their building. As soon as we were there for about 15 minutes, I had to guide everyone back down again, as Sabine's contractions became strong and steady. We went inside and I got things ready for the birth. Within half an hour her water broke and the baby came out.

And guess what! Dr. Margono was right. The cord was around the neck twice, but not tightly at all. If it had been tight, I could have handled it by cutting it, but I didn't need to in this case. I just gently lifted the cord over the baby's head once, then again, and he came out and breathed...well, beautifully. Sabine was on top of the world. She did it! I was thrilled, to say the least. And Ronnie was too.

By taking things one step at a time, unhurriedly, and by incorporating all of the parents' feelings—as well as those of the experts—we reached a great conclusion. *Yay!* One more unnecessary cesarean avoided because of excellent clinical management and great collaboration with doctors.

Recognition

~

Emily J. McGee, RN

Vinnie leaned over the nurses' station counter to say good morning. His easy grin radiated down from above me as I sat on the other side of the desk charting my morning assessments. His aura as chief surgical resident shimmered around him, glowing a bit brighter with his anticipation of graduation. I couldn't help but laugh at his obvious glee.

Our level 1 trauma center was firmly rooted in the ghetto—an oasis of hope buried in one of the most violent cities in the United States. The surgical intensive care unit had a taste of everything. Motor vehicle accidents, stabbings, and shootings were our soup du jour. Liver and kidney transplants our main course. It was, without a doubt, a harsh place to cut your teeth as a new resident, or a new nurse.

I had learned this quickly after the hellos and rushed introductions were made on my first day as a nurse. I went home with "If you can make it here, you can work anywhere," echoing off of my overly taxed brain, and against my skull.

The staff made sure I knew that orientation was the easy segment of my training. "Prepare yourself for the 'wolf pack,'" was repeated consistently during my first few days.

I soon cornered my preceptor away from the ears of the masses.

"What in the heck is the 'wolf pack?'" I blurted out.

He chuckled, seeing fear in my eyes.

"There are four nurses who have worked here for twenty years or longer. Jake, your preceptor on night shift, has been here for more than thirty. Jake knows her stuff, but won't give you an inch. Watch your back with her."

He leaned a shoulder against the wall, obviously enjoying my anxiety.

"Yup, they are all pretty opinionated. You've heard the phrase, 'nurses eat their own'? They take that mantra seriously. They have even been known to eat a resident or two, just for good measure."

That was all he gave me, and it was the only time I asked.

KNOWING VINNIE WAS scheduled for the ICU rotation was always a relief during my first year as a nurse. Not only did I trust his abilities, but I sat in quiet admiration as he approached patients in his calm, easy manner. He was an extreme contrast to many of the attending physicians he had trained under.

Many surgeons liked to blow through a unit, the center of a mini-hurricane of patient orders, scrambling residents, flying charts, and confused patients. Lights were routinely flipped on in the wee hours for hurried physical exams, and rushed conversations were normally held with patients who weren't given enough time to simply rub the sleep out of their eyes, let alone answer questions. Important discussions about their complicated hospital course were shrouded in complex medical lingo so the surgeon could keep control of the interaction, and not be hindered by long explanations. Most of the conversations were geared for the benefit of the residents regardless of the patient's questions or concerns.

Many times the nurse was left with the patient to apologize and offer medical lingo translations, all while reapplying dressings and recovering, at least part of, the patient's dignity. There is very little modesty for a patient.

"SO! HOW MANY days left?"

The question was thrown at Vinnie over my head. He had just come out of my patient's room where he spent more than a few minutes quietly discussing a surgical procedure with her and her family. He never hesitated to spend those few extra minutes to reassure a patient, or explain something, even if it was just explained a few moments before.

He lied. "I'm not sure. A few more weeks."

Vinnie knew down to the day. All of the chief residents did. Five years of grueling dues had been paid. They were each anticipating their new roles as attending physicians.

The nurse behind me chuckled. "Vinnie, you were such a pretentious ass when you were an intern!"

I spun in my chair to see who was asking, now able to see that it was Jake. Vinnie shook his head in the "Oh, shit. Here it comes" pattern that he was so good at. Vinnie was known for his playful teasing but always took it good-naturedly in return, especially from the nurses.

Jake had been on her way out the door, but stopped, continuing to pour on a bit more "don't forget where you came from" marinade. She also knew she had my attention.

"Oh, Emily! You should have seen him. He had an ego the size of a bus. Thought he knew it all! No nurse was going to teach him a thing. A regular, fresh out of medical school, know-it-all prick."

Jake was not known for her subtlety.

"No!" I somehow choked through my laughter directed at her insistence and his embarrassment. It was difficult to make Vinnie's dark complexion any shade of red, but she managed it beautifully.

Somehow, he missed—or did not listen to—the advice that senior residents traditionally pass on to the new interns: "Be nice to the nurses. They know more than you and will save your ass if you pay attention. They will make your life miserable if you don't!"

Although she sounded harsh, it was obvious that coming from her it wasn't chastisement. It was Jake's official public acknowledgment that he had made it. Without breaking into song and dance, spewing sunshine and roses, she expressed—for the first time in their professional relationship—that Dr. Mehta was finally worthy of a nurse's respect.

"Jesus, we had to break you. And, quite obviously, we did a good job of it too."

As quickly as she had started, Jake was finished. She gathered her bags, gruffly began complaining about something unrelated, and bumped the door plate with her elbow. Vinnie and I both turned and watched her go.

I glanced up at him.

"A pretentious ass, huh?"

"Yeah...well..."

He grabbed my patient's chart off the rack and began scribbling one of his last progress notes he would complete as a resident. I continued to laugh at his expense, knowing that the smile he attempted to hide was based on one of the hardest-earned compliments he would ever receive.

A Physician's
Definition of Failure

~

Mindy Owen, RN, CPRM, CCM

E<small>ARLY ON IN MY</small> nursing career, I worked
in large academic regional facilities. They were not
known as health systems then as they are today, but
as hospitals. We all know the kind of facilities I'm
referring to: The ones with teams of fellows and medical staff physicians who have practiced there for years,
and yet they are not the ones directing the day-to-day
care. That remains in the hands of the medical students, interns, and rotating residents who are writing
the orders and periodically asking the nurse if "that
order looks right."

As I look back on those days of nursing, in neuro-surgical-intensive care units, step-down units, and rehabilitation, it is obvious that in all we did to care for the sick and injured, we did it within the parameters of teamwork. From our day-to-day interaction, we knew each other's strengths and weaknesses. Physicians and nurses built relationships of trust and respect, so that in those crisis situations everyone knew their role and could be counted on to work together. It seemed like a well-choreographed dance—one leads and one follows and periodically the roles reverse and everyone under-stands that, through an unspoken creed.

After several years of working formally and infor-mally in roles as "charge nurse" on a variety of units, I was asked to work with a team that was developing a rehabilitation unit at a large regional medical center. This was to be a unit for patients with spinal cord or traumatic brain injuries. It would have a medical direc-tor who was a prominent neurosurgeon in the region.

I met with this neurosurgeon and discussed his vision and mine for this department. It was clear that he had the backing of this regional medical center and wanted to build a rehabilitation program for his patients and families to access and gain skills and knowledge that would not be available anywhere else in the state. He told me his role was to run interference with admin-istration; if needed, to provide medical direction and support, be the champion for the department with his peers, and enlist their assistance when necessary. But day-to-day operations, policy and procedures, program development, and support services would all be up to my team and me to implement. It was a challenge and commitment I chose to take on.

As the department evolved, we had a waiting list of patients who met the criteria and needed the services of this unit. We developed a process for admission and the medical director was always involved. He would participate in medical evaluation of candidates and give the patient and family a diagnosis and prognosis. He would then ask me to speak to families and provide them with information about rehabilitation. At times it felt like I was picking up the pieces.

Telling a patient's family that their loved one would most likely be in a wheelchair the rest of their life, or they would never be able to dress themselves, carry their child, or work the farm they loved was not an easy task. I didn't realize the emotional toll that those words had on this medical director.

I enjoyed meeting families—even in those difficult times—and felt that it was a big part of rehabilitation nursing to comfort, encourage, educate, and inform families and patients of not only what rehabilitation might be needed, but also to support them through the process. As I look back now, it was a division of labor between the medical director and me. He evaluated the medical condition and laid out the medical plan and I introduced the family to rehabilitation, evaluated their strengths and weaknesses, and formulated the plan of education and support. Oftentimes I would wonder why the medical director wasn't more involved with the families. I would always rationalize that he was busy with his practice.

This all became very clear to me one day on the unit when the medical director and I made rounds. We had an 18-year-old high school senior on our unit. He had been in a pickup truck accident and became a C6-7 quadriplegic. He was a wonderful young man, a good student, played varsity basketball, was a hard worker, and had been accepted to college. One stormy night changed his life. His pickup truck flipped over on a gravel road and he was left paralyzed. He had been in our facility two or three months at this point and was making good strides in his rehabilitation program. His personality was captivating and you knew he would find the positive in his situation and become successful in life. He had a supportive family and many friends that encouraged him through the program. At times I would tease him about having the "party room" on the unit.

One day when the medical director and I made rounds, I noticed that the patient's high school varsity basketball team photo was hanging in his room. He was an active part of the team when the photo was taken and he was standing in his uniform, in the center of the picture, smiling with all his teammates. I thought it was a great picture and I knew he was proud of it, as he had requested to have it displayed in his room. I called attention to the picture so that our medical director could see it. His reaction was one I will never forget. He stopped dead in his tracks, his face tensed up like I had never seen, and he nodded his head so as to acknowledge he saw the picture and abruptly left the room. I was dumbfounded at his behavior and followed him out into the hallway.

Once we were not around any patients or staff, he told me never to do that again. I was confused: I thought showing him the picture would give him more background about this young man and help the medical director understand who this patient is.

It did the opposite. The medical director told me that by seeing this picture it just confirmed that he had failed the patient. He could not give him back his life as it was before. He could not "fix" this patient, so in his eyes he failed him.

It was the first time I really understood the philosophy of some physicians—and the definition of failure to a doctor. I was shocked. Had it not been for this doctor's skill, talent, and vision of rehabilitation, this young man would not have the future he had in front of him. He would finish high school, go to college, get married, build a successful career, and have children. Why couldn't the doctor see that the patient had a future? It then became clear that my role as the nurse was to pick up the pieces and support the patient, family, and team. I wouldn't expect the doctor to carry that role.

After eight years of working with this medical director and building this department I resigned and moved to Chicago. As I was leaving someone asked why I thought we had built such a successful program. My answer was this: We all respected the skill set, talent, and expertise that each discipline brought to the program. The passion was something we all shared, but we knew that we all had a unique role to play and without each of us playing that role the patients and the program would suffer. No one discipline can carry a patient and family through the maze of medical care or rehabilitation: It takes professionals and staff, a well-oiled team that works well together. That doesn't come quickly or easily. It takes communication, talent, and commitment.

Failure? We didn't see failure on our unit, but the lessons we learned enriched our practice of rehabilitation medicine.

"Mistake, You Say?"

~

Bonnie Jarvis-Lowe, RN

DURING MY YEARS as an operating room nurse, I worked with an excellent anesthesiologist who had an ego as big as the universe itself. His argumentative nature was obvious and annoying to everyone he worked with, including the nurses, techs, and surgeons. No matter what the topic of discussion might be, he was always "right." His burning desire to be perfect at all times affected his temperament, as you might imagine—something we all ignored.

A discussion took place in the OR concerning a nurse who made a drug calculation error and gave an incorrect dose of medication to a patient. Her grief over the event was obvious and it saddened us to think about how she must feel. It was that conversation that caused the anesthesiologist to utter unforget-table words, words that remain connected to him to this day, even though he might have been right in his declaration.

"I have never made a mistake in my life," he said with a proud look on his face. Well, good for you, we all thought. He always seemed to voice those egotistical statements when we were not in a position to give a rebuttal. It drove the OR nurses right around the bend and over the edge. We were all type-A personalities.

One fateful day, when he was getting ready to do a general anesthetic, he mumbled something that sounded like, "I made a mistake."

The surgeon, surgical assistant, and five OR nurses turned and stared at him in total shock and awe. Did he say what we thought he said? He had a beautiful voice and was singing to himself as he pre-pared his medications for the day.

He suddenly realized what he had said and what was happening around him. Silence filled the entire room. He had to think fast in order to regain his composure, or lose his reputation as "World Class Egomaniac"—a title he cherished. By his expression, we knew the wheels were turning inside his head, as his eyes looked at no one in particular. After what seemed like minutes, he spoke the words for which he will forever be remembered. He looked at us with great pride, without blinking, and said, "I thought I made a mistake but my mistake was that I thought I was mistaken."

They're all still laughing! And so am I!

The Best Doctor
This Side of Heaven

≈

Angela Posey-Arnold, RN, BSN

MAKING ROUNDS ON my first full day as director of nursing (DON) in long-term care, one resident I talked with asked me if I was the doctor. I told her "No, ma'am. I am the director of nursing."

She said very honestly, "Well, I was wondering. I have been here for twenty years and I haven't seen a doctor yet."

That was my first clue that we had a problem.

Working in a 103-bed long-term care facility was all new to me. I had no idea of the massive world of the long-term care industry, but I had a feeling I was about to learn. The prior DON had taken all the books, records, and files from the office. I did not even have a job description. I was flying by the seat of my scrub pants.

I wasn't familiar with federal or state regulations, yet. But I did know good nursing and that is what I had to guide me.

I quickly discovered that the medical director, Dr. Nix, actually had opened the facility years ago and owned it for a number of years. He sold it five years before but remained as the medical director.

I worked with Margaret, a jewel of a licensed practical nurse. She administered medications and treatments with great skill and compassion. Margaret worked at the facility ten years earlier as a certified nursing assistant providing basic nursing care with ease. She worked her way up over the years to LPN and was now in nursing administration as infection control nurse. Margaret delivered nursing care with a pure heart of compassion. The residents loved and trusted her. I knew early on that she was the best right hand I could have hoped for. She told me that the DON had always met the medical director when he came on Fridays and that she would be with me the first time to show me the ropes. I observed as she went through the procedures of his weekly visit.

I was prepared to make rounds with him. When he came in, he went directly to the nursing administration office where an entire rack of charts had been rolled in for him. He sat down and proceeded to sign everything that had been flagged for him to sign. He never read one word of what he was signing. When he finished blindly signing everything, he asked if anyone was sick. Margaret reported who needed attention. He ordered meds and left. He never saw the first patient.

I thought, "This is okay: He knows all these patients and he will see them next Friday."

Next Friday he did the exact same thing. On his next visit, the following week, I insisted he examine four of our patients. I went with him. He walked in the room, glanced at the patient, wrote some scribble in the chart, and left. He was obviously incredibly irritated at me for making him see a patient.

I definitely had a big problem. I knew then the patients were not getting quality medical care. They were being neglected medically. I was terrified. We had Medicare Part A patients who were fresh from the hospital; they needed to be seen by a doctor. Most of them were only three days surgical post-op. Medical attention was critical to their recovery.

I had only been there three weeks when the state surveyors showed up. I had no idea who they were or why they were there. I soon found out who they were and why they were there. Frankly, I was glad to see them. I could tell by the panic on the administrator's face he wasn't as happy to see them as I was.

According to the survey, the facility had severe problems ranging from weight loss to pressure sores and overuse of physical and chemical restraints. The surveyors gave the facility 35 days to clean it up or they would be back to shut the doors. This seemed ominous, but it was a blessing because it started the ball of change rolling.

I knew there were some terrible problems and I was doing all I could to change things. But night after sleepless night I knew I couldn't accomplish this alone. The administrator stayed in his office all day and the nurses had been without leadership for so long that they too were flying by the seat of their scrub britches. Doing things the way they had always been done and not willing to change their ways. The surveyors did us all a huge favor—they got some attention and some action! I was only too happy to oblige them. I wanted the same things that they did—better patient care.

Corporate came flying in with all their weaponry like the cavalry. They sent in extra troops consisting of a registered dietician, occupational therapist, pharmacy consultants, and nursing consultants. I had a great clinical director and a wonderful teacher as a nurse consultant. Help had arrived and I felt relief.

The administrator was history. The new administrator and I spent five minutes together and knew that we were going to change this facility, beginning with the medical director. The problem was finding a new one before we fired the old one.

Amazingly enough, I had a sinus infection and went to see my doctor, Dr. Mack. His physician assistant (PA) saw me that day, and while he was looking in my ears, I had a thought: Dr. Mack! He would make a great medical director. He was kind, jolly, smart, and attentive. He had the help of a PA, and he had been a nurse before he was a doctor. He had the compassion and insight of a nurse and the authority and skill of a doctor. He was the perfect candidate. After discussing it with my administrator, I talked to Dr. Mack about it. He seemed interested.

Within two days, all credentials were checked and he was sitting in the administrator's office, ready to take the job. He was hired. We were happy. Then it dawned on me: Somebody had to fire Dr. Nix.

Dr. Nix had been the medical director for 25 years. There were two other sister facilities in that county and he was the medical director for all of them. He had been a doctor in that county for 30 years. Even so, he had to go. The facility needed a medical director and the patients deserved a caring doctor.

My administrator decided, to my relief, that it was her job to break the news to him. We waited until his normal visit on Friday. When Dr. Nix came in, there were no charts lined up for him and he was asked to go to the administrator's office. He rarely spoke to my administrator or me; I think we scared him.

She shared the results of the state survey with him. He had gotten a deficiency in most areas. That helped break the news. Then she told him that we were going to have to make a change and that he was being replaced. They worked out the details of the transfer of his patients to the new medical director and he left her office. Unfortunately, he came directly to mine. He walked in, closed the door, and chewed me up one side and down the other. He was angry, and he blamed me for everything. He threw a chart on my desk, ranted for a few minutes, and left. The words didn't hurt me and the chart didn't hit me, so I was fine.

WE HAD A RECEPTION welcoming our new medical director. He set aside one entire day a week to come to the facility. He came in, made rounds, examined patients, and cared about their well-being. I could call him any time I needed to and he wouldn't yell at me. We made things as easy on him as we could and worked together to turn the facility around from one with 35 level-A deficiencies to a model facility that provided a high quality of care and life. When the surveyors returned, ready to close the doors, they were pleasantly surprised at what the team had done in only 35 days. They said they could tell the difference as soon as they walked in.

Of course, they kept a close eye on us to make sure we were serious about providing quality care. The staff worked diligently, and in three years we had a survey that was very close to being deficiency-free.

Dr. Mack was the best the facility had ever seen. He really loved and cared for the residents and their families. They looked forward to him coming and they felt better cared for. It wasn't a burden to him. We actually talked him into playing Santa Claus at Christmas. He loved it. We loved it and our residents thrived. They thought he was the best doctor this side of heaven. Personally and professionally, I did, too.

Where the Heart Rules

~

Keith Carlson, RN

Working in an inner-city community
health center serving a largely Latino population can
be a dynamic and challenging experience, both personally and professionally. At the heart of this experience,
the nurse-doctor relationship plays a central role in job
satisfaction and personal fulfillment. Faced with inor-
dinate levels of chronic illness, HIV infection, teen
pregnancy, substance abuse, violence, and the lowest
per capita income rate in our state, the troubled yet
vibrant neighborhood that we serve is the platform
from which we operate. This particular health center
draws to it a special breed of doctor and nurse.

At the center of it all is a gentle giant of a doctor
who oversees the controlled chaos of the clinic with

an all-encompassing vision of community involvement and connectedness. Operating from this inclusive ideal, children, parents, substance abusers, the mentally ill, the chronically ill, the poor, the disenfranchised, and farmworkers — whether legal or illegal — are treated with equal respect and dignity. Despite its moments of relative dysfunction, the clinic hums along, serving thousands each week despite a no-show rate at times approaching 40 percent. The large number of overbooked patient visits and urgent walk-in appointments more than make up for the high no-show rate, and staff generally are overwhelmed by the multitudes who come rushing in the doors like waves breaking on a battered beach.

On any given day, we might see an elderly Hispanic woman complaining of chest pain, gesticulating and bellowing out in apparently grave discomfort, certain that she is on the brink of death. Later, after an EKG, nitroglycerin, a baby aspirin, and a medical evaluation, we learn that her grandson was arrested this morning on drug charges and her anxiety had simply gotten the better of her. Next, a middle-aged man struggling with addiction admits to selling his methadone in exchange for a night of heroin and debauchery, and now he comes to us, begging for Xanax and a shoulder to cry on. On his heels comes a pregnant teen, loath to have a baby, but religiously opposed to abortion. Her last baby is in state custody, and her mother lives on the streets. This is life in the healthcare trenches.

The medical director gathers talented staff into his midst, using the magnetism of his personality and his passionate vision of a just and righteous world to attract those who concur with his philosophy. Having cut his teeth as a young doctor during the heady days of the 1960s, radical politics and a mild but effective antiestablishment posture color his dealings with the powers that be. This Little Clinic That Could powers on, forging cutting-edge programs, often despite the lack of adequate staff, funding, and physical space.

From an outreach program for migrant farmwork-ers to a new paradigm in case management for low-income urban elders, the scope of programs grows from year to year. The clinic's success in reaching so many in this besieged neighborhood is often the fruit of stra-tegic partnerships with other neighborhood agencies, not to mention national organizations like The Rob-ert Wood Johnson Foundation and the Massachusetts Institute of Technology (MIT). The fuel for the clin-ic's engine is the director's stalwart dedication to the neighborhood's vulnerable populations, and his vision of culturally appropriate and sensitive healthcare.

Previously working as a visiting nurse assigned to this particular health center, I was apparently identified as a clinician who would be a good match for this clinical organism, and the medical director cast his hopeful line, drawing me in with patient persistence. Perhaps he recognized that my personality and clinical skills as a bilingual nurse with a sensitivity to the struggles of the urban poor would be a perfect match for the challenges at hand. Since that time, his method of mentorship has allowed me great breadth of practice with a firm knowledge that my autonomous clinical decisions would always be supported unconditionally, like restarting an AIDS patient on a previously prescribed drug he simply stopped taking, in order to protect him from pneumonia, or sending a patient to a specialist based upon my firsthand knowledge and clinical assessment. It is this power of trust and camaraderie that make this man, and the medical vision he has manifested, so compelling a leader.

One particular doctor with whom I have shared the management of many difficult patients at the health center is a man of great compassion coupled with incredibly keen clinical acumen. Bearded, with sparkling blue eyes, a quick laugh, and a demeanor unmatched in its kindness, he resembles a leprechaun among us mere mortals. Although his responsibilities often keep him away from his cluttered desk, his ability to focus, listen, and thoughtfully consider questions is one of his greatest attributes.

Whether we are sitting with a patient during a joint visit, conversing in the hall, or chatting amiably in a rare moment free of other distractions, what strikes me most is the level of respect that we have mutually created and nurtured in our relationship. It does not seem to make a difference that he has received far more years of training than I have. It seems pointless to consider that his superlative clinical skills outstrip mine by light-years (if these matters could be measured in such astronomical terms).

Despite the fact that my eleven years of nursing experience are easily eclipsed by his breadth of education, medical knowledge, and clinical experience, my questions and input are entertained with the same intensity of thoughtful consideration as are inquiries by his professional equals. In fact, when I am in his presence, I feel like an equal—and am treated as such—in spite of the ocean of experience and knowledge that separates us.

Still another physician comes to mind when considering the many superlative working relationships that I share with so many doctors at the clinic. This particular provider is another testament to the caliber of person that the director attracts to his side. Bespectacled, kind, clinically astute, outrageously knowledgeable while immensely compassionate, this provider, who sees both adults and children, brings a deep understanding of the struggles of families—especially those touched by AIDS, poverty, and violence—and she uses her knowledge of the psychosocial realms to augment the clinical work that we share.

Whether assessing a patient with AIDS whose disease is wreaking untold havoc on her body, or evaluating a family's ability to cope in the face of devastating illness and poverty, our mutually respectful and highly functional nurse-doctor relationship facilitates communication, puts patients at ease, and greases the wheels of a healthcare system that is often likely to repel even our most concerted efforts. There is an ease of mutual positive regard that infuses our conversations and interactions. When discussing a case, there is no palpable sense that one of us is more powerful than the other. We meet on a level playing field, and on that field nurses and doctors relate as colleagues without the encumbrance of hierarchy.

What I have learned in partnership with these outstanding doctors is that nurses, although often undervalued in outpatient settings, can serve in proactive, clinically meaningful roles if doctors willingly and consciously choose to utilize their specific skills and knowledge base.

In the context of this particular inner-city community health center, the majority of doctors—under the example set by a compassionate and visionary leader—

see nurses not just as handmaidens who only vaccinate children, refill medications, and dress wounds. These doctors come to this underserved and disenfranchised community in order to assuage many of the inherent health disparities that plague minority communities, and we nurses are part of this struggle as equal participants rather than unequal assistants.

When nurses, such as myself, are treated with respect by doctors, and doctors allow nurses a footing upon which to grow and learn alongside their cumulative knowledge and skill, magic can happen in clinical settings where lackluster medical care might have normally occurred. This community health center is not perfect—and some patients and processes still may fall through some significant bureaucratic cracks—but an underlying philosophy of mutual support and respect creates a clinical environment where I know that my input and skills are respected and wholly relevant.

Such a compassionate team approach to medical care pursued by doctors and nurses alike benefits everyone, and an entire community is uplifted in the process. This community health center strives for that idea—however imperfectly—and it is the nurse-doctor relationship that is at the heart of my personal satisfaction and our mutual clinical achievement.

Ms. Manners

~

Carolyn Lounsbury, LPN

"Get up and give that doctor your chair!" barked my nursing instructor, Mrs. Castle. She was an ex-army nurse and demanded that we take good care of our patients—and the doctors. She taught me to respect myself and my peers, which included the doctors with whom we worked.

In 1972, there were no surgicenters. Two mornings a week, I was the circulating nurse in a converted trauma bay in the back of an emergency room where we assisted surgeons with outpatient procedures. As a new grad, I was intimidated easily. On one of the first cases I assisted with, I was performing the five minute pre-procedure betadine scrub on an alert patient.

A gray-haired surgeon looked at the clock and asked sternly, "Can't you do that any faster?"

I looked at him dressed in a sterile gown, brown surgical gloves, fingers interlocked, rocking back and forth heel to toe. Flustered, I replied that I was doing my best.

"I've got other procedures to complete and I don't have all day," he shouted as he continued his dance routine. My face felt hot and my fingers began to shake.

"How can I do a five-minute scrub faster than five minutes?" I asked him.

"I don't know. But when you figure it out let me know," he replied. We had a good laugh and I never again let a doctor intimidate me. Through that experience, I realized that doctors are people, too.

THAT WAS 35 YEARS AGO. A lot of things have changed in medicine, but one thing is still the same: doctors appreciate a fresh cup of coffee after a busy night. They soften when you ask about their families and they're impressed when you express concern about the condition of a critical patient. If a doctor knows you care about him, he also knows you'll have the same respect for his patients.

Humor is my armor against stressful situations. When I worked on a telemetry unit in the 1980s, the on-call team was slammed with admissions: patients complaining of chest pain, rhythm changes like runs of V-tach, and myocardial infarctions. While a resident was in the emergency room with a crashing patient, an intern admitted patients. He came over to the nurses' station looking for the occult blood cards and liquid reagent needed for the rectal exam he was about to perform on a patient. Trying to help ease his stress, I sent him back to the patient's room and told him I would bring it to him. A nurse standing nearby reapplied her ruby red lipstick, opened the occult blood card and blotted her lips upon it. She was unable to contain her laughter. I delivered the two cards to the doctor along with the solution he requested. When he returned to our unit, I asked if the test was positive or negative. He answered with a big smile on his face that it had been very positive!

Throughout my nursing career, I have enjoyed working at large teaching hospitals. Each year, I anticipate the new batch of residents. I worry about the things they were *not* taught as I prepare to make them comfortable in their unfamiliar surroundings.

I ask them, "What medical school did you attend? Are you married?" Once I get them feeling comfortable, I test them just like I was tested. "What is the normal digoxin level?" With a worried look they confess they don't know the answer. I smile and touch their arm and tell them not to worry.

"Zero," I proudly proclaim! "I didn't say therapeutic level. I don't have digoxin in my blood and neither do you."

I hope to instill a sense of trust, respect, and humor for all the medical students, residents, and attending physicians who have crossed my path over the years. Surely they will remember the nurses who helped them write their first medical order, answered questions about doses, reminded them about appropriate medical tests for their patients, and made them feel at home with a much-needed cup of coffee. Perhaps one day, when we meet on a busy nursing unit, the doctors will return the favor, look my way and say, "Get up and give that nurse your chair!"

Smart Enough
Not to Be a Doctor

~

Pamela F. Gonzalez, RN

THROUGHOUT MY NURSING career, I have
heard the remark "You are smart enough to be a
doctor." This refrain has been voiced frequently by
patients, doctors, and colleagues alike. I know that it
is meant as a compliment, but it never ceases to bother
me. This backward compliment suggests that choosing a professional path in the nursing field is for those
with less intellectual abilities than those who chose to
go to medical school.

I want to retort, "Yes. I was smart enough—and
I chose not to be a doctor."

The choice not to go to medical school was not based on my intellectual ability. I have always tested well and been in the top of my class. In my undergraduate program at an Ivy League university, I studied alongside the premed students. In some of the nursing curriculum, I took classes with medical students and often set the curve. In my professional career, I have never viewed the physicians I work with as my intellectual superiors. I respect those who chose the path of medicine, and take every opportunity to learn from the MDs when possible. If my schedule permits, I attend grand rounds, journal club, and other educational opportunities.

The majority of my career has been in university-affiliated healthcare systems, and training residents and fellows. As a clinical specialist, I lectured in some formal training programs but the real teaching comes from the day-to-day interactions with physicians. Nurses are part of the check-and-balance nature of healthcare. MDs are human, as we all are, and sometimes make mistakes. The doctors I work with know that I don't page them about trivial patient care issues, and they come to trust my experience and professional judgment. I know my role in the healthcare continuum and the impact it has on patients. Most "smart" MDs appreciate the role of the nurses and value their collaboration.

MY NURSING CAREER has taken many paths, but my primary role has been working with HIV-infected and HIV-impacted patients. As an HIV coordinator, my relationship with patients was very different from doctors' relationships with the patients. I was privileged to have the time to teach people how to live with their disease: take their antiretrovirals, and thrive. I held their hands when explaining their diagnosis, spoke openly about risk reduction, and became an important person in their circle.

When AIDS first surfaced, in the 1980s, many patients felt stigmatized and socially isolated. I was someone they identified who could help them and stand by them without judging their behavior or lifestyle. Patients shared report cards, engagements, birth announcements, and other joyous milestones with me. I also was there when they divulged a drug relapse, or learned of a new opportunistic infection or a new STD despite the frequent frank discussions. I was there when they grieved over a lost partner or friend. I was there when a patient died and I was there at their funeral. Had I chosen to be a doctor, I fear that I wouldn't have been able to have this type of a professional relationship with my patients, and my life wouldn't have been complete.

Being a nurse means never having to say "that is not my job." Whether I'm collecting specimens, changing a dressing, or administering a painful IM shot, it allows me to be there with my patient—when they are most vulnerable. Nurses often are the cog that links all the healthcare pieces together: scheduling urgent doctor appointments, assisting with referrals and prescriptions, calling 911 to check on a patient at home, completing rent-subsidy applications, changing diapers, driving patients to rehab or shelters, delivering medications to their homes, and undertaking a myriad of other tasks. There is no job too big or too small that falls outside of the scope of a professional nurse. We help patients navigate the world of healthcare in a caring and nonthreatening manner. We are truly patient advocates.

In my experience, patients are more apt to provide accurate health histories to "their nurse" because they don't want their doctor to be disappointed in them. For example, during one typical HIV clinic day, after the patient saw his attending, he would meet with the HIV coordinator to perform a risk survey. When asked, during his history and physical with the attending, if he used condoms 100 percent of the time, the patient gave his doctor the "correct" response of "yes." Not more than 15 minutes later, when performing the risk survey, I probed further on his condom usage and learned that this patient always used condoms with his former wife, but never "with the skank that infected him." I then sent him for an RPR, a screening test for syphilis. I then spent the next three weeks administering IM Bicillin and focusing on risk-reduction behaviors.

Pursuing a medical degree most likely would have been a more lucrative path, but that certainly was not my priority. I was smart enough to know that choosing the medical path would mean years of training before ever interacting with a patient. I was smart enough to know that choosing not to be a doctor meant that HMOs and other entities couldn't mandate the amount of time I spent per patient. I was smart enough to know that choosing to be a doctor might prevent me from seeing the person in front of me as an individual rather than as just a diagnosis.

My choice not to become a doctor has permitted me a great deal of job flexibility. As a registered nurse, I have been able to work as a staff nurse, HIV coordinator, grant writer, travel clinic clinician, research coordinator, auditor, pharmaceutical sales representative, author, support group facilitator, ethics fellow, educator, and director of regulatory compliance. Regardless of my title, being a professional nurse has provided me with an identity and training that permits me the flexibility to fulfill career goals. I defend my "smart" decision: to become a nurse.

Rants to Raves

~

Kathy Quan, RN, BSN, PHN

N̲URSE-PHYSICIAN RELATIONSHIPS can be tenuous and many times they can make or break a career. This can lead to devastating effects on the severe nursing shortage. Throughout the world, many nursing associations as well as facilities are mandating improved conditions for nurses, which includes treatment by and relationships with physicians.

In any profession, those with the most power can either use it or abuse it. Physicians have tremendous responsibilities and therefore have to have a great deal of self-confidence. Unfortunately, this often leads to huge egos, even "God-complexes" or at the very least, arrogance beyond belief. In recent years, most doctors have learned to respect nurses as teammates, and patients as consumers who have a choice.

I'm a typical overachiever, and like most nurses, I strive for perfection in my patient care as well as administrative duties. We all know that this is not sustainable forever, and that errors will occur. Hopefully, they are few and far between, and of course not harmful or devastating to anyone.

In any given situation, I try to remain professional whether or not others are behaving in such a manner. I was taught that nurses who want to be respected need to respect others. That includes physicians—even the worst of them.

I remember one doctor who would stand at the nurses' station and yell, "Nurse!" I was a relatively new nurse back then and the delivery of care was different. There were no safe staffing rules and we worked eight-hour shifts. I was the charge nurse from 3–11 PM, the only RN on a 38-bed medical floor in a community hospital with one LVN to assist me. During a shift, we'd have as many as ten "total care" patients who needed to be fed and 19 or 20 running IVs—many of them hand-adjusted gravity drips. If we were lucky, we had a unit clerk, but many times only for part of the shift. I was expected to process orders and answer phones in my "spare" time.

So there was Dr. M shouting "Nurse!" The sound of his voice was enough to make me shudder. He was always so needy. I ran to see what he needed, and all he wanted was a pen. I reached to the right of him and selected one from the pile sitting on the desk in front of him. He sheepishly muttered something I took to be a thank you, and I went back to attending to patients.

The second time this occurred, I was in no mood for him. He was an older man, not some brand new hotshot doctor—he should have known better. We were short-staffed and the nursing office had pulled my second LVN out of the count to help on another floor with a higher acuity. I had just started an IV on dear Dr. M's patient when I heard him shout. The LVN and I quickly ran over to the nurse's station, thinking it might have been a patient emergency. He seemed pleased to have drawn such attention.

He dared to ask why there was never anyone at the desk; there was always someone available on the other medical floor—why was there never anyone here? He was pompous and indignant.

I looked at the Sue, the LVN, and sighed. I told him that there were two of us working tonight with 38 sick, needy patients. We have no unit clerk assigned to our shift, so I'll be processing orders and answering phones in my "spare" time.

I took a deep breath and asked what I could do to assist him. He looked at me with astonishment. His jaw dropped a little and for the first time, I thought I saw a glimmer of understanding. He was almost apologetic as he told me he had written orders on his two patients and wanted to be sure I could read them and that the charts didn't get overlooked because there were important labs to be drawn in the morning.

We reviewed the orders together and I set the charts on the absent clerk's desk. I assured him I would process his new orders as soon as I got a patient's IV started. He thanked me and asked me to please be gentle with her as she was very frightened of hospitals. Her husband had died recently and she had had a bad experience in that hospital. I didn't know that and thanked him for the information. That was important to her care.

I excused myself and went back to start the patient's IV. When I returned to the nursing station, I noticed him standing there and I worried that he was going to start shouting again. He walked over to the med cart, where I was gathering medication for a patient, and told me he was amazed at how much we accomplished on a shift and how well we worked together.

"It's obvious you care for your patients," he said with a smile.

We both learned a lot that night. He never again came to the floor and shouted, "Nurse!" He always alerted me to new orders in a patient's chart. And he always thanked me for taking such good care of his patients.

Our misunderstanding wasn't about making excuses or whining about the conditions of one's work, but more about communication and understanding our respective roles. I've found that if you're honest with physicians about the situation at hand, they usually come around. This usually diffuses the situation. Everyone has frustrations, and if something isn't right, work together to correct it. Mutual respect between doctors and nurses is essential to quality patient care.

The Nurse *Is* the Doctor!

~

Anna Gregory, RGN, BSc

I**N THE OLD DAYS**, nurses did their work and doctors did theirs. Somewhere along the way, the roles became blurred, and occupational nurses became responsible for duties once held by doctors.

I remember one of my first jobs in 1996 in Bromborough. I was sent to do a day's work performing lung function tests on employees exposed to flour dust. When I arrived, a lovely 76-year-old general practitioner met me at the door. He wondered why I hadn't arrived earlier in the day so that I could make him a cup of tea before the patients arrived.

As the day progressed I performed the pulmonary function tests. I then sent the patients to the doctor with the results. I wasn't allowed to interpret the results. God forbid that a nurse could do this!

Okay, I know this is very old-fashioned and that most of the employees did not need to see the doc with their lung function results. Around 90 percent of them were normal and I could have dealt with those patients. However, the employees went back to work pleased as punch that they had seen a doc and the managers were happy that their money had been well spent.

Fast forward ten years and we have gone from one extreme to the other. I did a shift a few weeks ago. When I arrived I was given a list of people on sick leave to contact. I called them at home and spent a long time on the phone with each of them. Many had complex illnesses, the details of which I struggled with. I had to use the Internet to look up some of the specifics about their diseases and prescription regimens before I could render any advice as to which drugs might affect their ability to drive or perform their job.

By the end of the day, the managers wanted a report from me, detailing how long these people were going to be off, if they were likely to come under the Disability Discrimination Act (DDA), and so on.

I found this difficult because in my other jobs, this was the doctor's role, not mine. As a nurse I was never taught these disease processes in such depth as to be able to estimate likely times of recovery. I am good at my job—I have a degree in occupational health (OH) nursing and 11 years of full-time experience. But I have always worked with a doctor.

I asked the company if they had a doctor. I received a blank look, and was told they used to have a doctor, but "the nurse is now the doctor."

I am lucky in that I have worked with an excellent OH consultant during the past ten years. When I was writing my reports to the managers, I visualized what the consultant would have said in the same situation. I managed to complete the reports and did a reasonably good job. The upshot of this is that the penny-pinching managers have won! They saved hundreds of pounds by using me rather than a doctor and I was stupid enough to do the work that they requested. I should have looked at them like they had two heads and said, "Actually, mate, this is the doc's job."

I know that many of my OH colleagues would criticize my views on this, but I am appalled that we are now doing the doctor's jobs. If for one minute I thought that we were being given these new roles because they thought we were an amazing group of nurses I would perhaps put a sock in it. But let's be honest here: *It's all about the money!*

I cost £25 per hour. The doc costs £150 per hour. Easy math. I agree that we can do much of the OH role but I also know where my competency ends and when to look to a doctor for advice.

My big worry is that when I have qualified as a doctor, which is the professional path I'm now pursuing, I might well want to return to occupational health. By then, though, there is a good chance that all the docs will have been replaced by nurses.

Grin and Bear It

~

Tilda Shalof, RN, BScN

Because i worked freelance for an agency in Canada, I was never in one hospital long enough to learn how things worked. Nights were particularly difficult because I had to figure things out for myself, such as when to call the doctor at home and when not to. Late one evening, I needed a laxative for one of my patients and I decided to page the doctor. She didn't answer, so after an hour I paged again. Finally, she called back.

"You're calling me now for that? You couldn't think of it earlier? I hate to think what you'd do in a code blue."

"Okay, I'll just chart *MD notified*."

"Oh, how you nurses love that phrase so you can pass the buck! Calling me about some trivial thing you could have figured out for yourself or just planned for ahead of time."

She was right. It *was* one of the oldest tricks in the book. Fobbing off my responsibility instead of merely speaking up for what my patient needed. But at that time, in most hospitals, a nurse couldn't even administer a laxative or a single Tylenol without a doctor's order. I went to my patient, but by then he was sound asleep and I wasn't about to wake him to give him milk of magnesia.

There were so many situations like that—where nurses' hands were tied. But most times, the stakes were a great deal higher than a laxative. Once, near the end of my shift with a mountain of charting still to complete, a call bell rang. It wasn't one of my patients, so I let it ring. "Let someone else go," I thought. But it kept ringing. I got up and went to answer it.

A man stood beside his bed, clutching his chest, face crunched in agony. "Oh, I've never had such terrible pain," he groaned. I placed an oxygen mask over his face and called for help.

"I'll get you a painkiller." I eased him down onto the bed.

"Don't leave me." He clutched at my arm. "I'm dying. Get my wife."

I felt his pulse. It was rapid and strong. "I'll be right back," I said and ran for the electrocardiogram machine. I pushed it straight out ahead of me as though it were a grocery cart and I was off on a madcap shopping spree. Running past the nurses' station, I called out for someone to bring me morphine and an aspirin because I thought he might be having an acute coronary event—a heart attack.

"The doctor hasn't ordered it," the nurse in charge said, looking up over her glasses at me. "He's in emerge right now, seeing a patient. Wait till he gets here."

But if I waited, it might be too late. I was not authorized to give a medication that wasn't ordered, nor could I administer oxygen without a doctor's order, or even perform an ECG without an order, but this was an emergency and I went ahead and did all of those things.

Later, when the doctor finally arrived and the patient was feeling much better, he was furious. "I didn't order this ECG!" he yelled at me and ripped it up. "Who do you think you are? If I report you, you'll lose your license."

It turned out the patient had suffered a mild heart attack as I had suspected, but it was hardly reason to feel vindicated. It was a serious setback for the patient, but what seemed to concern the doctor much more

was the possibility of a nurse threatening his authority. It was an old, unspoken, unwritten "doctor-nurse
game": You had to play and the rules stipulated that
even if you, the nurse, knew something, you weren't
supposed to let on. Diplomacy and tact were needed.
Suggestions or hints were okay, but taking action and
making decisions were far too bold. Even the nurse in
charge backed up the doctor.

"You are going to get yourself in trouble," she
warned, but did concede, "You may actually have
saved that guy's life. Maybe you really want to be a
doctor?"

"No, I want to be a nurse," I mumbled. But I
also wanted to be able to use my knowledge, skills,
and judgment. I hated knowing what to do and being
unable to do it; seeing things, but being unable to take
action. The worst was feeling invisible and unheard.

The medical docs were in it for the long haul,
were satisfied with small gains and took the inevitable setbacks in stride. They knew they couldn't fix
everything, but it was a darned interesting process to
try a little of this and a little of that and see what
happened.

On the other hand, surgeons were focused on
the bottom line, in "cutting to the chase," and in outcomes. They looked for opportunities to excise and
resect (remove and chop) or suture and anastomize

(sew and glue). They liked to fix the things they could—and quickly became disinterested in the things they couldn't.

Many doctors had favorite nurses and flirted with them, whether they were attractive or not. There were always a few who lived up to their stereotype, like the surgeon who showed up one busy morning needing help with a procedure he wanted to perform on my patient. "Hey, I'm putting a chest tube in Mr. Kanji," he said in an offhand manner. "He's got a pneumothorax and I may need a hand."

"And you would be...?" I asked as I continued preparing my medications.

"Hi, I'm Vince, from thoracic surgery." He extended his hand.

"Hi, I'm Tilda, from nursing," I said, mocking him ever so slightly. "I'll help you with that procedure as soon as I give the patient something for the pain first."

"Oh, he won't be needing it. The way I work doesn't hurt a bit."

"But he's already in a lot of discomfort from his surgery."

"Don't worry, he'll be fine. I'm very fast."

I bet you are. "But even so..." I recalled having read somewhere that pain is usually underreported, with pain medication under-ordered, and under-administered, and pain thus undertreated. I couldn't bear to think of doing that procedure—which involved making a deep cut into the chest in between his ribs, inserting a large, thick plastic tube into his deflated lung, and applying strong suction pressure once it was in place—without local anesthetic and a painkiller first.

"He won't need it," Vince said cheerfully, looking at his watch. "Can we get started?"

Oh, I get it. You don't want to wait while I get the keys and go to the narcotics cupboard for the drug. Then you'll have to wait a few minutes more for me to give it and for it to take effect.

"Don't worry," he cajoled. "I have superb technique." He patted me on the back. "None of my patients ever complain."

"That's because most of your patients are under general anesthetic."

"Aren't there any *nice* nurses around any more?" he teased, and I glared back at him.

Was it possible that he could really do such a smooth job that it wouldn't make a difference to the patient? Was I being over-conscientious? We stood on either side of the patient's bed and looked down at the man's emaciated body. I decided not to be on my side or the doctor's, just the patient's. I tried to fly inside his mind, so I would know what to do.

"Hey, is this guy even conscious?" Vince asked.

The patient had grunted and moaned a few times while we stood there but didn't seem aware of us, of our conversation or its meaning. "Anyone can see he's in discomfort," I said, and it was true.

"Okay, go ahead, give him something if it'll make you feel better."

I ran out and came back quickly with the drug. "Until this takes effect, there's the sink," I teased him. He hadn't even washed his hands.

"You're a pretty tough cookie, aren't you?" he said, grinning, donning a sterile cap and gown.

I hung a small bag of saline with two milligrams of morphine injected into it, but he didn't like this slow method. "Push it in, fast," he ordered, but I told him no: "I have to give it this way."

"But it will take too long to take effect if you do it like that."

"Even so..." Every patient reacted differently to narcotics—to all painkillers, in fact. For some, a small dose was enough to treat severe pain. For others with milder pain, a larger dose had little effect. Soon, the morphine eased our patient and the procedure went smoothly. Just before Vince left, he asked me out. I turned him down because first of all, he was a jerk, and second of all, it was around that time that I had reconnected with an old boyfriend I'd met in Israel.

Unfortunately, I didn't always speak up as assertively as I did that day. Once, after spending more than an hour on a complicated abdominal dressing that required rigorous sterile technique and deep internal packing, I had moved on to care for another patient when suddenly I head an angry voice in the hall outside the previous patient's room.

"Where's a nurse? I need a nurse in here right away!"

I ran back to find one of the staff surgeons tearing away at the bandages I had just spent so much time putting in place. "I need to have a look at this incision," he barked, ripping away at the tape and gauze pads and leaving the wound exposed. "Who did this dressing?" he growled. I swore under my breath as I stood watching him make a mess of my work. The patient seemed a bit bewildered but pleased to have his doctor there. "Would someone bring me a fucking pair of scissors?" the doctor shouted, right in front of the patient, and then glared at me—clearly the someone he had in mind. I scurried off to find a pair of scissors. It wasn't an easy thing to do, oddly enough, because each hospital kept supplies in a different place and I was always going on a scavenger hunt.

"Grin and bear it." A nurse said this as she passed me in the hall and saw I was upset. "We're nurses, aren't we?"

"Why do we have to take it?" I fumed.

"Don't let him get to you," she advised. "He makes everyone uptight, but he's a surgeon, you know. They get away with murder."

That remark made me giggle as I rushed back into the room, scissors in hand. But by then, the doctor was gone. He'd managed to remove the rest of the bandage by himself. The dirty gauze littered the bed and floor. The wound was left wide open. The patient's covers were thrown back and his gown was askew.

"How am I doing, nurse?" the patient, said, looking up at me. "The doctor didn't mention."

"Your incision is healing nicely." I was steaming mad as I repacked the wound with sterile gauze and then cleaned up the mess. On the bedside table, beside the chart, I found a fancy pen the doctor had left behind. He'd used it to write in the chart. It had gold-colored letters spelling out the name of a drug company. I did what anyone would do in that situation. I stole his pen.

Nurse Cherry Ames and Dr. Fortune Marry

~

Paula Sergi, RN, MFA

I USUALLY WAIT UNTIL I know someone quite well before revealing that I am married to a doctor. My reluctance to discuss my husband's profession is multifaceted and includes a Midwestern sensibility of modesty.

There's also the fact that I've lived through the second wave of feminism and like to believe that my own work is of greater interest than my husband's profession. I imagine that there was a time when the opposite was true; that women would readily announce their Mrs. Doctor status, savoring the prestige it afforded them.

Maybe it's because I'm a nurse and am biased, but these days I perceive a growing distrust and even disdain for the medical profession. The mere mention of the word *physician* brings up images of headstrong, bossy, egocentric people who have little respect for their coworkers. I know because I worked as a student nurse and staff nurse long before meeting my husband.

His career choice would have worked against him at the beginning of our courtship had his intelligence, warmth, ability to cook, and love of the arts not been immediately obvious. So it's hurtful to me to listen to grumbling and doctor-bashing; that is, unless the conversation addresses all aspects of healthcare reform.

There are quirky conditions that surround the doctor-nurse marriage. The most obvious is the quick mental leap to the stereotypical relationship made famous by novels from the 1940s and 1950s. Old concepts linger, and they are not flattering to anyone. Book covers featured a doctor looking lecherously at a pretty blond nurse. Remember Nurse Cherry Ames and Dr. Joseph Fortune? Despite her dedication and cleverness, she seemed to always be under his influence. The literature informing contemporary culture has promoted the notion that the most a nurse can hope for is to be the object of a male physician's lust. This bit of fiction masks the rich give-and-take that characterizes relationships between nurses and physicians, at work and at home.

Other ramifications are equally infuriating, like the situation I encountered one day when I was late for my son's sporting event and took a seat next to another mother. "I was working the immunization clinic," I explained.

"What do you do there?" she asked.

"I give the shots."

"Did your husband teach you to do that?" she wondered aloud.

Never mind my BS degree or ten years as a public-health nurse. The idea that just being married to a physician would allow me to be on the payroll of the local public health department infuriated me, despite my understanding that naiveté and ignorance were at the heart of that woman's comment.

Such ignorance is not wholly uncommon. We live in a small community and there's a weird curiosity about doctors' lives that hovers ominously. Though 40,000 people is not quite Andy Griffith's Mayberry, we have a large population at and above retirement age. Some really do listen to the police scanner as a hobby. When my husband was hospitalized for a kidney stone, the rumors included that he had suffered a heart attack brought on by my having left him. The convoluted facts about my husband's medical condition and the state of our marriage apparently were delicious to the hospital employees.

A weaker marriage would not survive the stresses that my husband's work has brought to our family. The number of meals we've had together in the last 23 years is minimal, because after a full day of hospital and clinic work, he returns calls to his patients and dictates his notes from the day. He also makes house calls to patients who are too ill to leave home or who are in the last stages of their lives. He attends his patients' funerals as a last gesture of care and respect.

People assume that the financial rewards compensate for evenings, weekends, holidays, and birthdays spent without my husband. The idea of being a physician's wife or child conjures piles of money at our disposal for all kinds of uses, and privileges galore. I know because I grew up poor and heard my neighbors, relatives, and the general public express these ideas in casual conversation and discourse.

Our children grew up knowing that their father's work took precedence, that he would be away long hours, and that bedtime stories, their sporting events, and elementary school performances were no exception. For a while, I worried about how this would affect them, but I was always aware of my husband's special warmth and of his ability to communicate his love and concern to our children. When I ask my now-young-adult sons about this they claim to have no resentment at all. "I always understood the importance of his work," they say, "and how he was helping people." They indicate that they might have resented his time away if he'd been on the golf course or playing cards or at a bar. But they knew he was always with sick people, and that was understandable to them.

My husband is not a saint. He has high expectations for himself and for those around him and these expectations sometimes are relayed in a shorthand that can be interpreted as critical. I have heard him ask a nurse to straighten the notepad messages in a patient chart because it is a legal document, and as such should not appear sloppy. This kind of attention to detail is not without merit but can be difficult to address when so many other tasks are pressing in a nurse's day.

As he ages, his perspective is becoming more rigid. He cannot understand his younger colleagues, whose primary concerns seem to be time off and salary. He is frustrated with the difficulties in attracting and keeping younger physicians in the internal medicine practice in which he is a partner. He has become intolerant of colleagues who do not hold or demonstrate good patient care as the gold standard by which they act and with administrators who haven't yet considered it, despite their lingo. He is tired of being called to wipe up the messes that surgeons leave behind. He is sad that his profession is all but lost, and blames physicians themselves for this sorry state.

Being married to a person who is totally committed to his work has its shortcomings. But it also demonstrates to our children the values of compassion, of a commitment to having high standards. It gives us a lot to be proud of. I don't have to mention this when I meet someone for the first time. Let them wonder about the person behind the woman who attends social functions alone and is not afraid to set the record straight about life as a nurse married to a doctor.

Laughing Too Hard
to Care

~

Heidi Lipka, RN

BEFORE I WENT to nursing school, I didn't really have any thoughts on what the nurse-doctor relationship might be like. Of course I had heard stereotypes about doctors mistreating nurses, but I think I believed in the back of my mind, well, it is 1995, surely those stereotypes don't exist anymore. Today, after having been a nurse for 11 years, I think that my belief was correct for the most part.

The majority of my interactions with physicians have been neither good nor bad, just benign verbal exchanges. I work the 3–11 shift in a small rural hospital where communications between nurses and doctors are over the phone or held briefly at a patient's bedside or at the nurses' station. Usually these events consist of nurses giving information to the doctor and the doctor giving or writing orders in response. On the other hand, the rare negative exchanges I have encountered—while few and far between—are the more memorable ones.

My first negative encounter with a doctor occurred while I was working as a medical-surgical floor nurse. I had just admitted a patient from the emergency department. I completed my nursing assessment and had written an admission note in the patient's chart describing my findings: Patient complaining of "right flank pain."

A short while later the admitting doctor called me over and asked who had written the note. I replied that I had.

He said, "The patient is having abdominal pain, not flank pain." Then he asked me, "Do you even know where the flank is?" I stared at him with disbelief. Was I supposed to answer him? Did he really think I could be that dumb? I pointed to my flank.

He proceeded to say, "That is not where the patient's pain is. It is in her abdomen; the note needs to be changed." He turned away from me, leaving me stunned and angry. I was still confident about where the patient told me her pain was and I did not change my note. It turned out that the patient had a condition that could easily cause abdominal pain or flank pain.

Another time when I felt mistreated by a physician, I was working in the same unit, but this time as charge nurse responsible for calling MDs with any important issues that might require immediate attention from a doctor.

It was around 10:30 PM and almost the end of an extremely busy and stressful shift. A two-day post-op abdominal surgery patient complained of chest pain. Even though we were confident that the pain was abdominal, the nurse did a set of vitals and an EKG. I called the surgeon to notify him of said chest pain, EKG, and the latest vitals. He had been asleep, which is never a good start to a phone call.

I relayed some of the info and before I could finish he interrupted me, stating he felt it was just GI discomfort, ordered Maalox, and hung up. After about 10 minutes he phoned back. Immediately he yelled into the phone, *Don't you ever call me to report chest pain without giving me vital signs!* He repeated this same sentence, again and again, not allowing me to respond. I became angry, but instead of yelling back, I started to cry.

I handed the phone to my supervisor, who happened to be sitting at the nurses' station but had no clue as to what was happening. I then walked away before the real tears came. Perhaps I was overreacting, but I was already stressed and the surgeon yelling at me was enough to throw me over the edge.

Having a sense of humor has helped me handle the subsequent, inevitable meetings with these particular doctors. What I do when I see one of them or if I need to call one is a simple visualization exercise. If you were a fan of the 1970s television series *The Brady Bunch*, you might remember the episode where Jan was nervous about speaking in front of an audience. Mike gave her the advice to "picture the audience in their underwear." She did this and ended up forgetting her anxiety because she was too busy laughing. I definitely don't want to picture any doctor I work with in their underwear, but for each one I came up with a funny visualization to help keep my nerves in check. I am too busy laughing, at least in my head, to let them get to me.

The first doctor, Dr. Youdontknowbasicanatomy, was fairly easy to imagine in a silly way. He is extremely short, round, and sports a decent-sized black pompadour. All I have to do is picture him in a sparkly white-and-gold jumpsuit (pant legs and sleeves rolled up) and *presto*—a mini-Elvis! This image can keep me smiling for a long time.

It wasn't hard to think of a funny image for the surgeon Dr. Yellsalot either. The fact that he seems to always wear a cowboy hat is funny in itself—for example, in surgery, while the rest of the surgical team stares at him, wondering, "Can that hat possibly be sterile?"

Fortunately, most of my interactions with doctors over the past 11 years have been unremarkable. I feel that these days, if a doctor is inappropriate to a nurse, we have the option of making a complaint without fear of retribution. So far, I haven't needed to. Is that because they have not been inappropriate at all or is it because I am too busy laughing to notice?

Everyone Cries

~

Cortney Davis, MA, RNC, APRN

"Untitled," by Jan F.

"I'LL TAKE CARE OF IT," the doctor said. And he took control. He had me touch my forefinger to my nose, walk a straight line and extend my hands. He delicately tapped my knees and ankles, producing uncontrollable jerks.

I was bled and photographed. Wires were fastened to my skull. Narrow sensors were placed inside my nose. My body was placed in a padded capsule, my head locked into place to obtain pictures of my brain. I didn't get to see any of the results.

"Good news," my doctor said when I reported back. "It's not a tumor."

"Oh," I said.

"What we have looks like idiopathic adult onset seizure disorder. Not uncommon," he said. "We have a number of approaches for controlling the seizures."

"Oh," I said.

The doctor prescribed pills. One the first day, two the next, three, then four. He would monitor the side effects. The tired feeling, nausea, and dizziness would pass.

"Get blood drawn and call in three months," he said, showing me out of the office.

The reality of the diagnosis rattled my settled life like an earthquake. Everything shifted. Impregnability was breached, control lost. Travel, jobs, friends, hobbies, sports, dreams—everything needed to be re-examined.

For the most part, I denied everything. As I stumbled through my drugged days, I pretended that I was still perched on bedrock. *The doctor will take care of it* was my mantra. I wobbled and spun, always tired or dizzy or nauseated. And I counted the days until I could report back to the doctor.

When I did, I would first surrender my arm, breathing deeply as the vacuum sucked my blood into tubes, sliding my eyes away from the diagnosis being written on each form. Trying to look normal.

"Things look good," the doctor said. "Your bloods are almost to the therapeutic level. Come back in three months."

Meanwhile, I worried whether each spell of indigestion or dizziness was the flu, the medicine, or a seizure. I called the doctor for reassurance. After I'd called a few times he sounded annoyed. I even felt foolish when I called to report another seizure.

He was brusque and replied, "We can take care of that."

I tried to believe his reassurance. *I needed* to believe his reassurance.

When I returned to his office, I had a chart plump with blood tests—stick figures with pluses and minuses over different areas—and reports of how electricity traveled through my brain.

"The bloods look good," he said. "We'll leave things as they are. Call me if you have another seizure."

My body continued to slip, losing its sense of harmony, until its only certitude was my ability to touch my nose and walk a straight line with my eyes shut. I gave up responding to unusual feelings, tried not to notice them, and certainly didn't bother the doctor.

I spent the next office visit crying over my losses. "It's normal," he said. "Everyone cries." But I was cautious in my tears, not wanting to say anything that would bring disapproval. And I didn't have the words for what the tears were really about.

When I started to cry during my next visit, he said: "More than once is unusual. Perhaps a psychiatrist?" and we returned silently to our ritual. Nose, reflexes, walk the line. Because I wanted to be normal in my abnormality, I locked the tears inside. And eventually I didn't feel them anymore.

I no longer owned my sleep, or my appetites. I felt my wit dull and my perceptions slow. Conversations seemed labored. I started rooting around in old diaries and picture albums. I wanted to find the real me from these snippets of the past, and then successfully rappel to the present, identity in hand.

I was unsuccessful. I couldn't separate age and change from disease. I felt lost.

However, I remained a compliant patient. Three-month visits widened to six-month phone calls. The side effects of the medicine were accepted, as was the occasional seizure.

My chart was filed under S for success. My bloods were correct, my neurological markers were normal, and I seemed emotionally stable. The doctor had taken care of it, as he said he would.

Hearing a Patient's Story:
A Commentary on "Untitled"

WHEN JAN F. WAS DIAGNOSED with epilepsy in 1976, her physician must have thought her the ideal patient. In the beginning, as "good" patients do, she let the doctor take control. She kept her appointments, took her medications, and tried to appear "normal" even when she "wobbled and spun, always tired or dizzy" from the drug side effects. But at some point, she stopped going to her doctor.

Jan F. wrote "Untitled" years ago, when she initially stopped seeing her physician. In her writing, Jan reveals exactly why she turned away from traditional medical care. She tells us what the initiation into the world of illness was like for *her*—a story we caregivers rarely hear.

What really happens when a patient receives a life-altering diagnosis? What happens when her acceptance of that illness doesn't jibe with the medical community's expectations? What happens when, in spite of her diagnosis, she *has things to do*, but can't talk to her care providers about how best to get on with her life?

In order to feel present, rather than ablated by her illness, she experimented with her medication dose and drank large amounts of caffeine. She became a psychiatric nurse and then a psychotherapist, often hiding her diagnosis from family, friends, and coworkers. She cleared trails for the Sierra Club, hiked at high altitudes, taught aerobics to seniors, and wrote poetry—seeming to have more energy, her sister told me, than anyone else her age. Jan F. lived her life fully until, on August 2, 2002, she suffered an epileptic seizure during the night and died. She was 61.

Reading this essay, I felt, viscerally, how difficult it was for Jan to be, suddenly, someone who must submit to testing, prodding, labeling. Her recording of conversations with her physician reveal the distance between them: His proclamation of "good news" and "It's not a tumor" didn't allow for the possibility that, to her, the diagnosis of epilepsy was bad news. The juxtaposition of her struggle with fatigue, nausea, and dizziness with the physician's comment, "Things look good," underline their disparate points of view: hers of a life forever limited; his of therapeutic blood levels.

When the specter of impending seizures hovers over "each spell of indigestion or dizziness," Jan seeks reassurance. When her doctor sounds annoyed, she feels foolish. When she cries, she's told, "That's normal." Eventually she locks her tears "inside" where they remained invisible to her provider. And when she at last assumes the mask she will present to caregivers for the rest of her life, her language becomes impersonal.

In order to survive within the medical system, she had to step back, out of herself. She seemed compliant, appearing to swallow both her medicine and her diagnosis. Her chart was "filed under S for success."

Though the focus of Jan's story is what the doctor did not do for her, for a variety of reasons, all of us may be similarly guilty. We are too busy to take time to listen to a patient; we don't feel comfortable dealing with a patient's emotional needs; we aren't qualified to deal with a patient's emotional needs. But what would happen, I wonder, if all patients wrote stories of their illnesses, and we had—and took—the time to read them?

Relinquishing a Soul

~

Terry Ratner, RN, MFA

At the moment you are most in awe of
all there is about life that you don't understand,
you are closer to understanding it all
than at any other time.

— Jane Wagner

I WATCHED A STRANGER'S heart beating today. It was the size of a fist, flesh-colored, and pulsating as blood pumped oxygen through his vascular system. I knew little about the man whose naked body lay before me, only that he had come into the emergency department four days earlier as a hit-and-run victim with a closed-head injury, two fractured femurs, multiple broken ribs, and a fractured right arm. His family said he wanted to be an organ donor and assist others in need when he no longer had use for his body parts.

One of the surgeons asked if I wanted to observe the procurement of organs. I thought about the recipients, somewhere, waiting for the delivery of a kidney or a liver. Were they dreaming of organs, packed tightly in ice, flown to their destination, to be transplanted in their failing bodies? I wondered if their thoughts weren't mixed with the sadness of losing a life to gain a life.

This was something new to me, as I worked as a nurse in the post-anesthesia unit and seldom ventured into the operating rooms. I hadn't viewed a surgical procedure for years and had never seen a beating human heart.

Two masked surgeons were gowned and gloved while one nurse filled out paperwork and the other set up suction and positioned the overhead lights. A surgical tech gathered shiny steel instruments and formed the sterile field around the patient.

The body on the gurney had been ventilated for the past four days. Calloused areas were visible on his feet and hands. He was a large muscular man, 35 years old, with a mole the size of a dime on his left hip. When I leaned in close over the gurney, I could see his pulse beating in the arteries of his neck. When I touched his arm, it felt warm and resilient, just like mine.

I watched as one of the nurses prepped his upper chest with Betadine and the surgeons prepared to cut. The man's lateral chest was discolored with purple and red ecchymoses, and his broken arm was bandaged with cast padding and Ace wrap.

The surgeon spread sterile towels that hid the patient's face, but from behind I saw thick strands of his long dark hair. Every few minutes my eyes wandered down to the coarse black hair that moved with the slightest motion. It somehow proved that a person was under the sterile blue cloths. I didn't want to see his face; that would have been difficult. It might remind me to look once again at the monitors that provided evidence of life—heart rhythm, heart rate, and oxygenation—proof that he was still living; not yet departed from our world.

The surgeon started to cut, as if unzipping a parka from the patient's lower abdomen up to the base of his neck. Then, with a sharp instrument, he sawed lengthwise, so that the rib cage could be parted, before installing a large retractor that pulled the two sides of the incision apart. Now it was as wide as it was long.

Dressed in blue scrubs, a yellow isolation gown, and a mask, the surgeon held an electric cauterizing wand. It looked like a cheap bank pen on a cord but functioned like a scalpel. The wand cut and burned as the surgeon made his incisions, melting shut each severed vessel, causing less bleeding and an odor like seared meat.

Even on the inside, the patient looked very much alive. I watched the pulse of his heartbeat in his liver and all the way down to his aorta. The electronic beat from the heart monitor reinforced the impression that the patient was a living, breathing person.

I thought about my science class in high school and how I had dissected frogs. Some of the girls had giggled and turned red, but I'd wanted to take part in the dissection and learn about their anatomy. I used sharp blades to carve out organs and set them on a blue towel before labeling. I watched the delicate hands of squeamish girls unable to cut through the slimy skin. Boys laughed to cover up their feelings while slicing their frogs into cubes. The ambiguity I felt then was with me today.

In college, I remember the cats, all different sizes and colors, waiting to be dissected by eager pre-nursing students. Then there were the cadavers, a man and woman who donated their bodies to science so that nursing students could probe and use scalpels to dissect each organ. Somehow it seemed easier to work on bodies that were cold, stiff, and discolored than to observe organ procurement. I knew the cadavers were dead, more like rubber mannequins than humans, but the man on this gurney had soft skin, with some color to his face, and his symmetrical lungs moved up and down with equal breathing—inspiration and expiration.

An anesthesiologist stood behind the hidden face, watching the monitors and regulating the patient's oxygenation. The hum of the ventilator, the beats reverberating on the screen, and the click of the staple gun blended in with Billy Joel's greatest hits playing on the stereo. I stepped up on a stool to view the opened chest and stared at the amazing muscle, the human heart, counting the beats and watching the synchronized movement gently lift and fall. It's a mixing-machine part, the human body's most animated organ.

The patient had hepatitis C, and transplanting his heart was not an option. I was told that a recipient wouldn't last a year with his heart, but his kidneys and liver would be transported to someone in need.

I watched as the surgeons carefully examined his liver, turning it side to side and noting the healthy color and size. They said it would be sent to California for a hepatitis C recipient. One of the donor network nurses explained that people with hepatitis C share the same body chemistry, and so a recipient with hepatitis C adapts easily to a hepatitis C donor's kidney and liver.

I stared at this brilliant creation, thinking about God's creatures and my heart, your heart, the hearts of all the staff in the room. I've heard that when surgeons take out a heart for transplant, the room becomes silent, prayer-like. They say that once you hold the human heart in your hands, you'll understand that feeling. It's like holding someone's soul.

The lungs were striped with black lines from smoking, and I wondered what those tar-damaged organs might have looked like in 30 years. The intestines were as long and amazing as I remembered them, a coiled labyrinth of machinery perfected by the same creator. One of the surgeons bundled them together under sterile green towels, as they continued to suction and do their work.

The abdominal and thoracic aorta had to be crossed-clamped before the kidneys and liver could be removed. I watched as the heart muscle quieted, as the fast dance became a slow waltz. It quivered a bit before it stopped its movement. The anesthesiologist turned off the monitor and ventilator and left the room. His work was finished.

A dose of Heparin was given to prevent clotting, as a nurse poured crushed ice into the abdominal cavity. The surgeons suctioned out blood before procuring the liver and kidneys.

The differences between life and death became issues in my mind as I tried to understand the organ donation process. I thought about the spirit and soul and wondered what the difference was. I'd always felt the soul to be in one's heart. I wanted to pinpoint the precise moment when the spirit, the soul—whatever you wish to call it—has ceased to exist. This very body that looked only bruised an hour ago began to turn a darker shade with a tint of blue and had a hardened, cold exterior. I knew the look of death. Before my eyes, the body had discernibly altered. Something—call it spirit, or soul, or life force—had departed. I heard myself sigh deeply, as though, with his departure, I too had been freed. The quandary of that thin line between life and death was no longer there.

I thought about a soul's passing. *Do departing spirits fly by loved ones, brushing against them in noticeable ways? Do they hover over their useless bodies, procrastinating over their fate?* I'd heard many stories. A patient in the recovery room told me she had once died in a previous surgery and was brought back to life.

"I was above my body, looking down at the chaos taking place in the surgical room. Then I was in the waiting room watching my husband and family cry in a corner. I knew the time wasn't right to die," she'd said. "When I recovered, my heart and soul were somehow changed. I saw things in people I never noticed before."

We looked at one another and held each other's hand. We both understood.

But this body lying before me wasn't going to recover. His soul and spirit must move on. Is there a special heaven set aside for people who die like this?

I listened to the sound of my own breathing, felt the puffs of breath that circulated around my blue mask. I breathed in and breathed out. For a moment, I felt lost even within the area around me. I looked across the room and imagined all of us with that miraculous muscle pulsating, keeping us alive, that familiar sound reverberating in my ears when I place my stethoscope on someone's chest: *lub-dub, lub-dub, lub-dub*. We were here, my coworkers and I, still part of the material world, our souls still somehow, somewhere attached to our bodies, perhaps to our hearts. Rays of light seemed to radiate through the room, past the man with long, dark hair, past the surgeons and nurses. And I knew a man's soul had moved on.

Acknowledgment of Permissions

"Please Help My Son Not Die" is reprinted with the kind permission of Nancy Leigh Harless. The story originally appeared in *Womankind: Connection and Wisdom Around the World*, released by Tate Enterprises October 2007.

"A Truth about Cats and Dogs" is reprinted with the kind permission of Adrienne Zurub. The story is adapted from her memoir, *Notes from the Mothership: The Naked Invisibles*.

"Grin and Bear It" is excerpted from *A Nurse's Story* by Tilda Shalof © 2004. Published by McClelland & Stewart Ltd. Used with permission of the publisher.

"Everyone Cries" is reprinted with the kind permission of Cortney Davis and Sondra Zeidenstein. It is based on the story "I'll Take Care of It" by Jan Feldman and originally appeared in *Stories of Illness and Healing: Women Write Their Bodies*, edited by Sayantani Das Gupta and Marsha Hurst, Kent State University Press, 2007. Jan Feldman died in her sleep in 2002 of an epileptic seizure. Feldman was a mother, a psychiatric nurse, sculptor, writer, mountain hiker, windsurfer, and high-energy gardener. In addition to having a psychotherapy practice, she facilitated cancer survivor groups, provided counseling to incarcerated adolescents, and taught yoga and exercise therapy to community groups.

Reader's Guide

1. Nurses and doctors are expected to work closely together as they jointly strive for the well-being of their patients. Should institutions be accountable and committed to establishing and maintaining environments that promote excellence in the nurse-physician relationship? What principles should be included in a Professional Code of Conduct?

2. The nurse-doctor relationship is often at the heart of a healthcare institution, as Keith Carlson writes about in "Where the Heart Rules." How has the working relationship between nurses and physicians affected you, whether as a nurse, a physician, or a patient?

3. Nursing requires in-depth education, intense training, and expert judgment, not unlike the training doctors undergo. However, this often is overlooked by those outside the career who have misconceptions about the field of nursing. How

has this inaccurate view of nursing affected nursing school enrollment and the nursing shortage? What has the media done to promote the role of nurses? What can be done to create an accurate view of the nursing profession?

4. There's much more to being a healthcare professional than simply understanding anatomy and medication: It takes compassion, too. In "The Best Doctor This Side of Heaven," Angela Posey-Arnold writes about how one doctor's "softer" skills affected the nurses, staff, and patients in her facility. How have the physicians you know been able to combine knowledge and compassion? Describe some ways hospitals might bring compassion to the bedside for both residents and nurses.

5. Mindy Owen writes about the necessity of a well-oiled team. How has the team environment among nurses, doctors, and staff affected your own work, if you work in the healthcare field? Discuss ways to improve teamwork within an organization. As a patient, working his or her way through the medical maze, what impact did teamwork have on your experience?

6. Perceptions about nurses and about doctors may well affect how we interact with one another, as Nancy Leigh Harless describes in "Please Help My Son Not Die." Think about perceptions—or misconceptions—you have had about the doctors with whom you work. How have those perceptions affected your working relationship? How has a "negative" first impression of a colleague impacted your working relationship? Describe a strategy which might alleviate misconceptions about healthcare professionals.

7. Stereotypes about the nurse-doctor relationship abound, as Paula Sergi describes. How do stereotypes affect your career as a nurse? Or your experience as a patient? What has been done to break down these stereotypes?

8. The nurse-doctor relationship can be a challenging one, and many have complained of being ill-treated by doctors. But sometimes, all it takes, as Carolyn Lounsbury writes in "Ms. Manners," is a smile, a pat on the back, or a kind word. Think about a time when a doctor treated you with professionalism, respect, and kindness. How did you react? Did that event affect how you treated your colleagues? Your patients?

9. Patient care is a partnership and takes teamwork, communication, expertise, and compassion. But not all patients survive. If you are a nurse, think about the short and long-term effects after losing a patient. Now, consider how that same loss affected the doctor with whom you worked on that case. How did that experience change the way you practice nursing? As a patient, or a patient's family member, how have you seen nurses and physicians react? What are the similarities? What are the differences?

10. Nurses often are expected to show initiative and offer advice while at the same time deferring to a doctor's authority. Sometimes this requires refusing a doctor's orders, as Karen Klein wrote about. If you are a nurse, think about a time when you had to consider this option. What were the circumstances and how did you handle the situation? When it came to charting the refusal and reason, what steps did you follow and why?

11. In "Home Delivery," Cara Muhlhahn writes of the misconceptions many people have about midwifery. What misconceptions does she recount both from the patient's perspective and from the perspective of the medical community? How does

she work with physicians to create a partnership that is satisfactory for all involved?

12. Nurses often spend a considerable amount of time with patients—sometimes much more than doctors do. As a result, nurses frequently have insight into patient care that a doctor might not have. If you're a healthcare professional, think about a time when you believed you could add a crucial ingredient to improve a patient's care. How did you articulate that insight? At your last visit as a patient, how long did you spend with nurses and doctors? What type of care did you receive from each person?

13. As more men enter the field of nursing and more women become doctors, the typical female nurse/male doctor stereotype has shifted accordingly, although perhaps slowly. How has this evolution affected your own career? Or your perceptions as a patient?

14. "It's easy to get lost in the poetry of medical words." So writes Cheryl Dellasega in "Every Patient Tells a Story." Medical professionals often work in stressful environments which may cause them to value their own words over those of the

patient. Think about a time when you or a physician impacted a patient's care by focusing on the "art of listening." Discuss situations where you were able to preserve the person in the patient. As a patient, remember a time when you felt you were, or were not, listened to by your healthcare providers.

15. Adrienne Zurub writes that most "surgeons acquire a 'distancing' veneer in order to do the necessary work." If you are a nurse, discuss your experiences in an operating room setting in which, as Zurub describes, "Arrogance, entitlement, outstanding talents and confidence dominate the entire operating room suites." What are some of the communication techniques that allowed you to work in this environment? If you have been a patient in an OR, how did the surgeon distance himself or herself from you? How did that affect you?

16. Nurses and doctors are often too busy to take the time to listen to their patients. Cortney Davis says in *Everyone Cries*, "We don't always feel comfortable dealing with a patient's emotional needs; we aren't qualified to deal with a patient's emotions." Davis takes the focus one step further when she questions what would happen if all patients wrote

stories of their illnesses and nurses and doctors took the time to read them. Think about a time your patient related a negative story about his or her healthcare experience. What was your reaction? As a patient, describe a time when you tried to communicate your feelings to a nurse or doctor, but they were unable to focus on the emotional aspects of your concerns.

17. Improved communication, doused with respect, humor, and understanding between doctors and nurses leads to better patient care and enhanced patient outcomes. In Heidi Lipka's *Laughing Too Hard to Care*, she says having a sense of humor helps her to handle confrontational doctors. What are some strategies nurses can adopt to foster better communication in the workplace? Discuss why a zero-tolerance policy for disruptive behavior and verbal abuse is paramount to addressing this type of conflict.

18. Ending the anthology with Terry Ratner's *Relinquishing a Soul* brings up important issues of life and death and the integration of science and God. "They say once you hold the human heart in your hands, you'll understand that silent, prayer-like feeling. It's like holding someone's soul." Nurses

often have conflicting thoughts about prolonging life for various reasons. Discuss a time when you had conflicting feelings about a doctor's plan of care. How did you address your differences? How do we keep our cultural and religious beliefs from interfering with patient and family decisions?

About the Editor

TERRY RATNER, RN, MFA, is a registered nurse, freelance writer, and creative writing instructor. Ratner's nursing career has spanned more than 17 years at Banner Good Samaritan Medical Center, a level-one trauma hospital in Phoenix. As a longtime advocate of positive nurse-physician relationships, she has researched and written extensively on the subject for national nursing publications, including *NurseWeek* and *Nursing Spectrum*.

Ratner teaches creative writing in a variety of settings from community colleges to a school for homeless children (Thomas J. Pappas) to wellness communities throughout the Valley of the Sun. In 2004, she launched an Arts and Healing program for children undergoing dialysis. Ratner is a strong proponent of clinical narratives, the writing of stories to assist nurses in understanding themselves and their practice. She has won awards in both national and local nonfiction competitions. Her writing has appeared in *Johns Hopkins Nursing*, *American Nurse Today*, *eHealthcare*

Strategy & Trends, Today in PT, Raising Arizona Kids, Phoenix Magazine, and *The Jewish News of Arizona.* She lives in Phoenix, Arizona. www.terryratner.com.

About the Contributors

KEITH CARLSON, RN, is a registered nurse who practices in New England. An avid writer, his work can be found at several blogs: www.digitaldoorway.blogspot.com, www.latterdaysparks.blogspot.com, and www.treonurse.blogspot.com.

CORTNEY DAVIS, MA, RNC, APRN, is the author of three poetry collections, most recently *Leopold's Maneuvers* (University of Nebraska Press), and a winner of the Prairie Schooner Poetry Prize and the American Journal of Nursing Book of the Year Award. A memoir about her work as a nurse practitioner in women's health, *I Knew a Woman: the Experience of the Female Body* (Random House) won the Center for the Book Non-Fiction Award. She is also co-editor of two anthologies from University of Iowa Press, *Between the Heartbeats: Poetry and Prose by Nurses* and *Intensive Care: More Poetry and Prose by Nurses*, winner of the American Journal of Nursing Book of the Year Award. Cortney's collection of essays about the art of nursing is forthcoming in 2009 from Kent State University Press. She has received an NEA Poetry Fellowship, three Connecticut Commission on the Arts poetry grants, and three Pushcart Prize nominations. www.cortneydavis.com

CHERYL DELLASEGA, PhD, is a prepared nurse practitioner and professor in the department of humanities at Penn State College of Medicine and in women's studies. Her clinical work has focused on psychosocial issues, particularly as they relate to women. Dellasega is the award-winning author of six commercial nonfiction books and a young adult fiction series, and has won awards for her poetry and short stories. She is the founder of Club and Camp Ophelia.

PAMELA F. GONZALEZ, RN, received her bachelor of sciences in nursing from the University of Pennsylvania School of Nursing. She completed graduate work at the University of Illinois at Chicago and is presently undergoing a Bioethical Fellowship at the MacLean Center for Medical Ethics at the University of Chicago. Her primary interests include HIV patient advocacy and improving the quality of conduct for clinical research.

ANNA GREGORY, RGN, BSc, has wanted to become a doctor since she started her nurse training in 1992. It took her 10 years to get around to applying to medical school, and in the meantime, she spent many happy years working in occupational health. She is married to a teacher, and she is in her third year of medical school.

NANCY LEIGH HARLESS, NP, has had stories included in many anthologies including *Cup of Comfort*, *The Healing Project*, *Chicken Soup for the Soul*, and *Travelers' Tales*, as well as many professional and literary journals. A graduate of Intercollegiate Center for Nursing Education in Spokane, Washington, she worked largely in the area of maternal child health before receiving her advanced degree, as a women's health-care nurse practitioner.

BONNIE JARVIS-LOWE, RN, is a 59-year-old retired registered nurse who worked in various hospitals across Canada. She retired at age 51 to return to her home province of Newfoundland and Labrador with her retired policeman husband. She has been practicing and enjoying her homeland, photography, and writing since retirement. She has two adult children and one grandchild in western Canada, and misses them terribly. Travel looms in the near future.

KAREN KLEIN, RN, is a magna cum laude graduate with a bachelor of sciences in nursing from Adelphi University. Her varied nursing experience includes ER/trauma, pediatrics, interventional radiology, telemetry, ICU, home infusion, and occupational health. She is a certified emergency nurse and an AHA CPR/first aid instructor, and has been published by *Nursing Spectrum Magazine*.

HEIDI LIPKA, RN, has been a registered nurse for 11 years. She has worked in the medical-surgical department in a small rural hospital in Vermont for the last seven years. She is the author of the blog *Green Mountain Country Mama*, where she writes about being a nurse, mother, and wife.

CAROLYN LOUNSBURY, LPN, has worked as a licensed practical nurse for 35 years at Level 1 trauma teaching hospitals in Arizona. She has interacted and indoctrinated hundreds of rotating residents throughout the years and continues to use etiquette and humor as teaching props.

EMILY J. MCGEE, RN, MSN, APRN-BC, NREMT-P, is a flight nurse at Aero Med in Grand Rapids, Michigan. She is also a nurse and captain in the U.S. Army Reserves, and works as an emergency room nurse practitioner. In her spare time, McGee writes about flight nursing at www.crzegrl.net. Her hobbies include anything involving massive amounts of adrenaline.

CARA MUHLHAHN, CNM, BSN, practices full-scope midwifery in a private practice setting in New York City. Her previous experience includes the Maternity Center, Inc., and Beth Israel Medical Center, both in New York. Her work has been featured in *Parents* magazine and the *New York Times*. "Home Delivery" is excerpted from her forthcoming memoir, *Labor of Love*.

MINDY OWEN, RN, CRRN, CCM, began her career in healthcare as a critical care specialist in neurosurgery and rehabilitation. She was a charge nurse of a neuro ICU and step-down unit at Milwaukee County Medical Complex. She then joined the team that designed, developed, and implemented a SCI-TBI rehabilitation at Wesley Regional Medical Center in Wichita, Kansas. Owen was the first regional director of CM for Intracorp. She is a Charter Board member of CMSA and was its second president. Owen has served numerous local, state, and national boards and organizations, including the CMSA, CCM, and ARN. She is an advisor for several publications, journals, and pharmaceutical companies. Owen is the Principal of Phoenix Healthcare Associates, LLC, a consulting firm specializing in education and development of case management and disease state management programs.

ANGELA POSEY-ARNOLD, RN, BSN, is a published Christian author and retired RN, living with her husband of 20 years in a log home in beautiful northwest Alabama. Her writing and music studio, Pebble East Studios, is located in the loft of the log home. Posey-Arnold has been widely published, with two Christian nonfiction books, many short stories, Christian articles, devotionals, and poetry. Her work also has been featured in *Faith Writers Magazine*, and she is a regular contributing writer for the popular e-zine www.4Him2U.com. Her newest book is *The Nightingale Protocol*.

KATHY QUAN, RN, BSN, PHN, has been a nurse for more than thirty years. After a few years of hospital nursing, she pursued home healthcare where she worked as a field nurse, a nursing supervisor, and a quality improvement specialist. She is the author of four books including *The Everything New Nurse Book* and writes for several websites and blogs such as TheNursingSite. com.

PAULA SERGI, RN, MFA, was selected by the Hessen Literary Society as the Wisconsin writer to act as the 2005 Cultural Ambassador for the Hessen-Wisconsin Writers Exchange and received a Wisconsin Arts Board Artist Fellowship in 2001. Her poetry is published regularly in such journals as *The Bellevue*

Literary Review, *Primavera*, *Crab Orchard Review*, and *Spoon River Poetry Review*, and her writing has been featured in the *American Journal of Nursing*. She holds an MFA in creative writing from Vermont College and a BSN from the University of Wisconsin, Madison. Formerly a lecturer in the English Department at the University of Wisconsin, Oshkosh, she teaches creative writing at Ripon College. She worked as a staff nurse at University of Wisconsin Hospitals, as a public health nurse with various county departments, and as a visiting nurse in Portland, Oregon.

TILDA SHALOF, RN, BScN, is an intensive care unit nurse with twenty years of experience in Israel, New York, and Canada. Her first book, *A Nurse's Story: Life, Death, and In-Between in an Intensive Care Unit*, was a bestseller that received rave reviews.

ADRIENNE ZURUB, RN, MA, CNOR, is a speaker, comedian, actor, and poet. She is the author of the bestselling memoir *Notes from the Mothership: The Naked Invisibles*. Formerly, she was on the Cleveland Clinic open-heart team for more than twenty years. Adrienne enjoys sleeping, Internet surfing, and waiting for something magical to happen. Her blog can be found at http://adriennezurub.typepad.com.

Meditations *on* Hope

Nurses' Stories about Motivation and Inspiration

~

Paula Sergi, BSN, MFA
Geraldine Gorman, RN, PhD

EDITORS

COMING TO STORES IN OCTOBER 2008!

Julia
(or the Burden
of Bearing Witness)

~

Keynan Hobbs, MSN, RN

JULIA CAME BACK TODAY to the unit, where I work as a psychiatric nurse. The story that is passed among the staff is that this time she checked into a hotel in a manic state, bought almost $800 worth of food and crammed it into the kitchenette, and after a week caused a scene that brought the police.

I ask her how in the world she had spent $800 on groceries.

She says angrily, "They were staples!"

The attending and resident assigned to Julia decided to file for conservatorship for her because she has been in the hospital so often in a short amount of time.

She asks me, "Why can't I just go back and live in the house I'm paying for? That I own half of? That my family takes advantage of me to live in? I gave up a life of my own to buy that house!"

I ask her what she means about giving up a life of her own, but she doesn't respond. She's not keeping eye contact now, sitting with her hands folded in her lap, and starting to cry and rock back and forth. I think she is now somewhere far away from where this conversation started. She says, "My mother told me that house would always be mine!"

When Julia starts to talk about her mother, a bright red hue creeps up her neck and face until it overtakes her whole head. It is remarkable against her white hair. I give her chances to regain control on her own, then I do a grounding technique that brings her back to the present and the red tide slowly recedes until Julia is not happy, but at least isn't shouting, crying, and clenching her fists. She recounts to me how she was abused as a child. This isn't the first time she's told me about this, but it isn't any easier to hear than any of the other times. I get her some medication. I used to avoid using medication to help her calm down, because it made me feel like a failure and because when it is offered, Julia will often say mockingly, "Oh sure, Julia, here's more medication, take it and shut up!" I went one shift with her insisting on only using verbal intervention; I really gave it my best. And it was good—but not good enough. It only put her on a roller-coaster ride of calm and rage: up and back down, up and back down, up and back down. Now when I give her the medication and she starts with, "Oh sure, here's more medication..." I just tell her that she isn't being fair.

Later, Julia wants help mailing her nursing license renewal. This has been an issue between us because she believes that I should see her as a peer, but I can't. I see her as too ill to practice, but she insists that she isn't. I can see and appreciate the nurse in her, in how she organizes our linen closet, in the volunteer activities that she tells me about, and in how she handles her medications—but I think I see it because she works so hard at showing it to all of us. She says it is evidence that she isn't sick—that everyone else around her is the problem, not her. But her actions are always tempered in some way by her mental illness: They may be nursing in spirit, but are no longer nursing in form. It is as though her judgment is simply gone, and that stands out as a significant reason for why I can't see her as a peer. I think that I will have to be clearer in my own mind about what a nurse is—and can be—before this conflict will be resolved.

IT IS TIME FOR A meeting with Julia's mother concerning the home they own together. When we enter the room, Julia sits across from her mother. I sit roughly between them at the end of the table, next to a social worker and a physician. Julia's mother is in her eighties and has a stone-faced affect. After brief introductions, the stage is set for some big news from Julia's mother: She states—slowly and matter-of-factly—that when the papers were drawn up to make Julia part owner of the home, the notary in attendance was a friend of the family and never intended to file the papers. Julia has never owned half of the house; telling her that she did own it, her mother says, was "to give you some sense of self-esteem."

Julia screams, "But I gave up my life to buy that house! I paid half of the down payment! I put on new windows, a new roof…"

Her mother denies that any of this happened, though she won't keep eye contact while doing it. "Any money that you might have paid into the home was rent as far as I'm concerned," she says.

Julia screams back at her about the years of abuse she endured

"Julia, you are like a dog," her mother says, and she looks straight into Julia's eyes for this. "You are like a dog that has broken through thin ice and lots of people are all coming out to you ... and we can either let you drown or hit you over the head and save you."

BACK IN JULIA'S ROOM, she is still bright red, screaming, crying. She sits in a chair, hunched over and yelling, and pounding her clenched fists into her thighs. As she yells, I think about starting a grounding exercise for her, but I don't. I think about getting medication, but I don't. Instead I kneel down and I put my hand on hers, a boundary I ordinarily might not cross, but just for a moment I put my hand on hers and I witness her suffering. I'm stripped bare by what I've seen today, and all I have left to offer her is to bear witness. And, as Julia begins to quiet, I'm pleased to find that a witness is, in fact, exactly what she needs to get through this moment and on to the next. Julia allowed us to connect enough to get through this moment together, and that leaves me with hope that healing is still possible.

As a psychiatric nurse, I am often privileged to see the most personal and private parts of a patient's life. I may be the only person they can talk to about something, because I may be the only person in their life that isn't part of its cause. The incredible risk that comes with this is taking the stories in—and having no way to let them back out again; then they become a burden. I have many techniques that I might apply to any situation, but two appear to be essential for me to ease suffering and make positive change when it matters most: the ability to take in another's suffering and the ability to let it back out again.

When the Patient Becomes the Teacher: A Lesson in Hope

~

Dorothy Consonery-Fairnot,
MSHA, RN, CCM, CLNC

Have you ever thought about how suddenly your life can change? I am a workers' compensation nurse case manager. The most challenging case of my career came when I was assigned to work on a catastrophic case involving a 23-year-old male who received an electrical shock while working on a construction site. By the time I was assigned to the case, Jim had undergone several surgeries as a lifesaving measure, which resulted in the removal of half his body (a hemicorpectomy).

This case was transferred to me when Jim was three months post-injury. Upon arriving on the ICU burn unit, I was greeted by the ICU case manager, who discussed the case in full and gave me an opportunity to read Jim's extensive medical record. The evidence was clear that although Jim had survived an accidental electrocution, several surgeries, and infections, he was not out of the woods yet. His condition was listed as stable but critical. My initial responsibilities included assessing Jim's medical, psychological, and social needs and condensing them into a comprehensive short- and long-term treatment care plan with a goal of having him reach his maximum level of functioning. Having to establish a long-term treatment goal was quite challenging based on Jim's condition and because the medical survival rate for such patients was poor. Based on these factors, I realized that to make the greatest impact on this case, I would have to use aggressive case-management interventions to maximize Jim's chance of recovering from this devastating injury.

Upon entering Jim's ICU room, I was met by his father, a man of small stature with eyes that cried out for answers. He could not speak English, but I knew the questions he—as a parent—must have: Why my son? Will he live or will he die? Will he be an invalid for the remainder of his life? I gestured to him and tried my best to explain that I was there to help his son. The father's nod let me know that he understood that I was there to help. I knew then that all of my future visits would require a professional interpreter.

Jim lay motionless in bed but opened his eyes once; clearly he was medically sedated to allow his body to heal from the sheer physical shock of losing so much of his body mass. Imagine the impact of a multisystem body trauma: There are so many deficits that your body has to learn to compensate for that. It is no wonder that few survive this type of body-mass loss. But Jim was alive—and fighting.

Make no mistakes: his physicians were amazed that he was still alive, but they did not give me false hope. His chances of survival and full recovery were poor.

I visited Jim weekly while he was in ICU and I spoke with the ICU case manager several times during the week. To everyone's amazement, Jim's medical condition was improving day by day. My patient survived ICU and spent another nine months in an inpatient rehabilitation center. He gained use of his left arm. His right (dominant) arm had to be amputated, disarticulated at the shoulder level. In total, Jim spent more than a year in a hospital setting being nursed and rehabbed back to a full medical recovery. The numbers of major and minor surgeries he endured were countless—let's say more than 20, including several skin grafts.

Rehab taught Jim how to strengthen his left arm and how to make this his dominant arm. His upper body became very muscular and strong enough that he was able to use the overhead trapeze bar to pull himself up while in bed.

Remember, this young man now had half of his body; his surgery included a disarticulation at his hip level. He could not turn himself, but he learned how to roll over by himself. He was fitted with a thoracic bucket to fit into his wheelchair.

Jim surpassed all expectations and triumphed over every obstacle. Above all, he did it with such human dignity, becoming an example to all who worked on his multidisciplinary team. Jim had the courage, wisdom, and ability to see that self-pity meant defeat—and that wasn't a part of who he was.

As professionals, we were challenged by his decision not to accept sympathy: life had much more to offer than feeling sorry for him. We were cautioned that Jim could become depressed. I remember one group session that included his psychologist, who reported that Jim was not showing signs of depression but that she wanted him to remain on the antidepressant medication. Depression could cause a major setback in his treatment. I was thankful that that day never arrived.

During his care on the rehab unit, Jim's psychologist found a church-affiliated hospital volunteer group that taught English to non-English-speaking patients. In one year, Jim went from uttering a few words in English to speaking and understanding the language very well. He learned how to paint landscapes; I have the two pictures that he gave me hanging in my office as a reminder that true courage can lead you to a greater place.

My goal was to transition him from a rehab facility into a handicapped home setting. I was faced with many challenges in my collaborations with everyone who was involved on his case, which included attorneys, adjusters, employers, and several physicians. I cannot stress how important it is to develop trusting relationships with all parties involved on your case, conveying a central message that you are a nurse advocating for the best medical care on behalf of your patient.

In the course of arranging for Jim's discharge home, I arranged for a handicapped van and for him to attend college to learn computer graphic art. What a joy it was to see him go to college. He was so excited and he talked and talked about the other students he met.

Jim was very fortunate in that he had a father and sister who relocated to this country to take care of him, which allowed him to remain in close proximity to the physicians who saved his life. Jim's family was truly a major support system and a testament to his longevity by providing him with love and excellent home care. With a good family support system, even the severely injured individuals have been known to increase their life span.

During the course of four years that I managed this case, I experienced so many emotions. I was taken to another spiritual level by my interactions with Jim. I had never seen such real hope, courage, dignity, humility, and strength—and it came from someone so young.

There was a bond between Jim and his physicians that I had never experienced in 25 years of nursing. I felt it when I was in their presence: they were a team who fought this fight together and they won. I heard physician after physician tell my client's story: someone greater than us spared his life so that everyone who encounters him will see hope and love of life in action.

Is there a greater gift for humankind than this? Jim never lost hope, never became depressed or angry. Instead, he was an inspiration and lesson in compassion and hope for all who had the privilege of treating him.

Mr. Bunyan

~

Madeleine Mysko

A<small>FTER HIS WIFE</small> died, he sold their home and moved into an apartment in our independent living wing. Already he was in trouble: congestive heart failure, edema, shortness of breath, and nasty skin eruptions in places he couldn't reach when he bathed, which wasn't often. Moreover, there were unexplained scrapes and bruises—evidence he'd suffered a couple of falls, though he vehemently denied it. He should have been packed up and moved to the healthcare center weeks earlier, where he would have received the nursing care he needed. But he wasn't the sort of man anyone just packed up and moved.

He was in trouble, and we both knew it, but only one of us was going to admit it. That would have been me: the "new" nurse recently graduated from the RN refresher course, the one cheerfully determined to deliver the very best practice in geriatric nursing, the one he consistently addressed as "lady," as in "Ask you something, lady—do your people ever communicate with each other?" or "Listen, lady—nobody's going to pull the wool over these eyes."

He was a big man. I'll call him Paul Bunyan, because sometimes when I visited him—when he was still able to draw himself to full height—he'd tower over me like the fabled lumberjack. Also, he had a favorite flannel shirt that he wore year-round—red, a lumberjack plaid.

Once upon a time, Mr. Bunyan applied his engineering acumen and his big, capable hands to overseeing the maintenance of an entire complex of university buildings. But age and sickness put an end to that. And so he wasn't as good-humored as the storybook character. Sometimes he could be really mean. I would walk the eighth-floor hall toward his door, brace myself, and pause to take a breath before lifting the knocker. Though he'd never really threatened physical violence, on more than one occasion he'd slapped the wind out of me with his swift and stinging sarcasm.

Mr. Bunyan's apartment certainly wasn't the largest to be had in our retirement community, but I imagine it was the largest he could afford, and he was proud of it. The living room was good-sized, but, unfortunately, it appeared rather cramped, like the way a fresh new apartment always does when too much dark, heavy furniture from the former home is forced upon it.

By far, the best feature of the apartment was the balcony beyond the sliding glass doors, with its view of downtown Baltimore and the Inner Harbor. On a clear day, one could see the distant Francis Scott Key Bridge glimmering over the bay. Mr. Bunyan was particularly proud of that view. Sometimes, in the midst of arguing with me, he'd suddenly change the subject to that view, sweeping his big hand toward the sliding glass doors like he was lord of it all: open air, lots of it, carrying the weather over the roofs and treetops of the city—a silvering of snow, the sweet clarity of spring, the oppressive heat that Baltimore is famous for in the dog days of summer.

And then, of course, he'd return to the arguing.

Mostly we'd argue about whether Mr. Bunyan was really in trouble, alone in that apartment. I saw trouble aplenty: he was weak and getting weaker; he was vulnerable to falls, noncompliant with his diet and medications, and embarrassingly remiss in his personal hygiene. I was tactful, of course, in making my case.

Mr. Bunyan's opposing view was that he could manage just fine, if only I were more efficient in providing nursing assistants who could "get the job done"—bathing and personal care, housekeeping, laundry, meal preparation, medication management—in the few hours a week he'd allow them in. Mr. Bunyan was not particularly tactful in making his case. He referred to my staff as *your people*, as in "Your people never arrive on time" or "Your people have got my pill boxes all mixed up" or "Listen here, lady—tell your people that the food in my refrigerator belongs to me and I'll throw things out when I'm damned ready."

A more experienced and confident nurse would have quit arguing sooner. But I had just returned to nursing after years away. A divorce had borne down on me like my own personal tornado, leaving me bereft of purpose in my life. I coped by pinning my RN badge to my freshly ironed uniform jacket and striding out on rounds in my sensible new shoes. To each of my elderly charges I'd bring sunshine and sympathy and hope that things would turn out all right, if for no other reason than my appearance in their apartments. I was their good nurse, their true advocate.

Of course, it was vital to me that the residents liked me. Just about all of them did. All but Mr. Bunyan. He would have none of my advocating for good nursing care. Instead, Mr. Bunyan made me his adversary.

A more experienced and confident nurse would have quit the arguing simply because of the obvious:

inevitably, Mr. Bunyan would be wheeled out of the apartment in full-blown heart failure or suffering from either a fractured hip or a fractured skull, in which case neither of us could be declared the winner. My fear, of course, was that one day I'd knock and hear no irritated bark of reply, that I'd have to let myself in to find he'd died, alone, but sitting right where he wanted to be: in his recliner, the TV tray before him with its mess of half-eaten food and pill boxes, that stunning view of Baltimore behind him. No doubt Mr. Bunyan would have counted that one a win.

In the end, Mr. Bunyan did move to the health-care center. As irony would have it, he moved when I was off for a few days, and so we both were spared the awkwardness of facing each other at such a sorry time. But remarkably—or perhaps this is the rare instance when "miraculously" applies—this story really ends some time earlier, on the day Mr. Bunyan and I achieved our truce.

It was a summer day, hot and humid outside, but unnaturally cold indoors with the air-conditioning blasting like a nor'easter. I could have used a sweater as I made my rounds, and it made me feel peevish that I felt so chilled all through the chaotic workday.

In my pocket I was carrying a list of nursing feats I could no longer imagine pulling off. In the back of my mind I was carrying heartache: the house in which

I'd raised my children was up for sale and I was trapped in the letting go, unable to even step into the backyard where my cherished perennials—lilies and cosmos and black-eyed Susans—were now in bloom.

And so I knocked on Mr. Bunyan's door that day with my mind made up to take whatever blame he was prepared to heap on me, to bear up under the strain, to smile and back away—anything to get out of there without losing my grip.

As for Mr. Bunyan, he was having an inexplicably good day. He had only one complaint: that I kept sending him "new people," though he allowed today's "little gal" seemed nice enough.

"Look at that beautiful day out there, will you, lady," he said, changing the subject, looking over his shoulder toward the view.

It wasn't a beautiful day. Beyond those sliding glass doors, the sky was gray with oppressive heat and haze, probably working itself up to a summer storm.

He frowned, studied my face. "Bad day?" he asked.

I pressed my lips into a smile. Suddenly, I couldn't speak, couldn't look him in the eye.

"You ought to step out there and take a breath of fresh air," he said. "It'll do you good. And while you're out there, why don't you pick yourself one of my tomatoes."

I slid open the door and stepped into the heat of Mr. Bunyan's balcony.

He had moved his sickly houseplants out there and someone had filled the window boxes with red geraniums. In the corner, leaning out through the railing, was a leggy tomato plant on which were ripening no more than a half-dozen tiny tomatoes.

He had said "one," so that was what I allowed myself: one small tomato, the size of a gumdrop. It was warm in my hand, firm. I held it carefully while I took in the view of the city. Thunder rumbled in the distance.

"Did you pick yourself a good ripe one?" Mr. Bunyan asked when I stepped inside.

I held it out for him to see—one small, ripe tomato, still warm from the sun, centered in my palm. "I'm going to save it," I said. "A treat for my lunch."

"You'll find it's sweet," he said. "Almost like dessert."

Afterward, going down the hall, I kept my hand in my pocket, still cradling that tomato. But later, alone in the elevator, I withdrew the tomato and placed it in my mouth. It was sweet indeed—a sort of communion, an offering of peace, hope that everything would be all right.

Final Moments
Nurses' Stories
about Death and Dying

~

Deborah Witt Sherman,
PhD, APRN, ANP

EDITOR

*COMING TO STORES
NEAR YOU JANUARY 2009!*

House Call

~

Cortney Davis, MA, RNC, APRN

Even from my position at the doorway I could see that he was clearly lifeless, a blank look replacing his usual grimace. His wife had been calling the office all afternoon, every half hour, then every fifteen minutes. The last call had been one of sheer panic. "I can't wake him up," she said. "I think maybe this is it. Please. Please come right away."

A nurse practitioner, I'd been making house calls to Mr. Cardone for months, examining him at home when he was unable to come to our office. I'd seen him through his surgery, his radiation, and then the last-ditch chemo that didn't cure him but only made him melt, it seemed, until every week he became a smaller, frailer version of himself.

Now, his wife's anxious voice, her *I think maybe this is it*, told me that he was most certainly dying. I knew that Mrs. Cardone, although expecting this moment—almost wishing for this moment—was not, now that the moment had arrived, sure she could endure it. And so I rushed through my last patient visit of the day and quickly drove the winding back roads to the Cardone's brick house on the lake. The late May day was lovely—the trees still in their new-spring green—and I couldn't help thinking that it was, perhaps, a good day to die: better than a cold, iced-in day in January; better than a rain-soaked, windy day in April. When I pulled into their driveway, I saw Mrs. Cardone appear briefly at the window, waving me in. In a moment, I was standing at the open screen door.

Her husband, Martin—"Manny" to his friends and family—was lying on the couch, face up, arms folded over his chest as if he were napping. He was dressed in fleece pajamas, too heavy for this warm day but the only clothes that could keep him from shivering, could keep his thin legs and veiny arms from trembling. He had one slipper on; the other had fallen to the floor.

Mrs. Cardone now stood in the far corner of the living room, looking not at him but at me; beside her, almost hidden behind her skirts, stood their granddaughter, Rebecca. Even during these days of illness, this time of distress, Manny and his wife continued to care for six-year-old Rebecca while their daughter worked. What, I wondered, had Rebecca seen and heard, living so close to her dying grandfather? Like her grandmother, Rebecca looked not at Manny but at me. Both of them seemed afraid to move closer to him, afraid even to cry for him—knowing, and yet not really knowing—that he was gone. Somehow, I was needed to make this official: a verified death; the end of a forty-nine-year marriage and the end of a long and cumbersome illness.

This wasn't the first time I'd gone to someone's home, making the house call that made official what the family suspected. Every time had been different and yet, in some ways, every time had been the same. I'd learned how to go slowly through the motions of checking the pupils, hollow and staring; of listening for heart sounds and hearing only their strange absence; of auscultating lungs that did not rise and fall, automatically, as they had for a lifetime. As I leaned over Manny I could hear, in the background, the sounds of a washing machine, the hum transmitted through his chest to my ears. Perhaps Mrs. Cardone, eager to maintain some sort of routine, unable to stop to contemplate the lack of momentum that is death, had done some laundry. Perhaps she asked Rebecca, as a distraction, to help her.

I'd also learned, in all the times I'd bent, silent, over the dead, that there are few words necessary to confirm the fact that death has actually occurred. It only takes a look up at the family, a brief *I'm sorry*. These words always draw the family in, closer to the bodies of their loved ones, as if, before, there had been something fearful there, something not quite alive and yet not certainly dead. Somehow, those two words allow the family to move past fear, past that awful suspension of time, into the here and now. Now, someone is dead. Here, there are things to be done.

Mrs. Cardone moved to stand beside me and I hugged her, put one hand on her head to guide it to my shoulder. I reached down and put my other hand on Rebecca's hair, stroking it. As Mrs. Cardone sobbed, I looked beyond her to the deep blue lake and the equally azure sky. At the base of their yard, a small dock reached into the water. A rowboat was tied there and, in the breeze, rocked back and forth, with a faint, repetitive *clink*, on its tether. I wanted to reassure them that the body is only a brief container; that Manny had gone to a better place—and yet, at that precise moment, I couldn't imagine anything more heavenly than what he had just left behind.

Dabbing her eyes, pulling herself together, Mrs. Cardone's resolve seemed composed equally of relief and anger, robbed as she was of the man who had partnered her through more than two-thirds of her life, robbed even of the daily routine that had occupied her for the months of his illness: the bathing, the trips to the hospital, the giving of medications, the nights when he would sleep fitfully, grunting for breath, and she would not sleep at all. Rebecca, dry-eyed, pulled at her grandmother's skirt and demanded a stop to this grieving and help with coloring, a bunch of crayons in her fist—a six-year-old, eager to divert all this onto the pages of her coloring book where she could scribble and scratch the sadness away.

Mrs. Cardone straightened. "I'll call my daughter," she said, then knelt and whispered into Rebecca's ear, scooting her into the kitchen. Next, she directed me. "Call the visiting nurse," she said, "and let her know there's no need for the aide to come tomorrow. I don't want her to make a wasted trip." The death moment, the hard realization, had just passed. We all got busy.

Manny's daughter arrived in the doorway, hesitating, taking in the scene. Mrs. Cardone, the strong one now, held out her arms. "Come to me," she said. "Dad's gone." While they wept anew, I called the visiting nurse who said, "It's about time. I thought he was going to hang on forever." Then I went into the kitchen to sit with Rebecca.

While Mrs. Cardone and her daughter murmured and talked in the living room, calling friends and neighbors, making the necessary arrangements that keep one from breaking down, from smashing one's fist into the wall, from taking to one's bed, I sat with Rebecca, who said, "*Now* we can color." I colored the birds blue. She colored the flowers and the vines purple and red. She chatted to me about nursery school and about the swimming lesson she had taken the day before. Death seemed a thing as yet unable to touch her. I wondered if she had a doll somewhere that might later need dressing and feeding, those pretend ministrations and tendings that would prepare her in some way for a day, far in the future, just like today.

I stayed in the kitchen with Rebecca until the funeral home came to collect Manny's body. His wife and daughter watched as the hearse pulled away; then Rebecca and her mother took Mrs. Cardone upstairs to pack a bag—she would stay with them for a while—and I walked out to my car. As I drove away, Rebecca waved to me from the bedroom window, and I waved back. In a moment she disappeared, but I could hear her as she ran back to her mother and grandmother, laughing, innocent, and alive.

The Changing of
the Seasons

~

Terry Ratner, RN, MFA

THERE ARE TWO main seasons in Phoenix:
summer and winter. Our fall and spring are bypassed
for long stretches of sameness. Maybe there's a hint of
spring in March, when a frail rain falls casting a silver
net over the neighborhood. Then the sky clears and
the flowers smell like baby lotion until the aroma is
suffocated in blazing heat. These are our seasons.

Nursing also has its own seasons. They follow no
direct weather pattern and occur as suddenly as a hur-
ricane or earthquake, without any warning. There are
brief periods of calm with little activity, just the daily

comings and goings of patients—the ones who recover without much pain, without any scars.

Then the changes occur: trees with still branches begin their dance; the full moon wears an orange veil as winds throw blankets of dust like confetti up toward the sky. In daylight the air fades to sepia, like an old photograph. That's when code bells chime and intensive care units fill to capacity with dying patients and grieving families. The scent of loss is everywhere and one can't escape the inevitable season of death.

It begins in the arteries, rushing sounds without words. Some agree, "It's too soon for death." And others welcome the freedom from pain. The season of loss passes by like a series of cold breaths.

THE WAY I PRACTICE nursing might have been different if I hadn't lost my mother in the spring of 1993. The time of year when the nights stay cool and days begin to warm. That's when I began to bond with little old ladies wearing turquoise rings, silver earrings and glittering beads. I'd hold their hands and laugh with them like old friends. I'd study their faces searching for a connection: hair the color of freshly fallen snow, skin paper-thin, eyes shining like topaz, and a dimple on the left when they smiled.

My nursing care changed again in the spring of 1999, when my son, Sky, died in a motorcycle accident.

All the young patients became a part of me—each one taking up a small space in my heart trying to fill the emptiness. They brought about poems of music, stanzas without metaphor, making something out of nothing.

It all happened during the season that's sometimes missed. During the season that hides; the one that smells like jasmine and sprouts tulips from the darkness of the earth. A season that cools the evening sky with its sweet resinous wind while orange tree petals drift to the ground like snow. The season filled with colors; fairy dusters with pink puffs radiating from their centers and clusters of purple wisteria trailing their vines around budding trees. That's the season when my world caved in.

Those deaths affected my career in ways I never understood until now. They left a sickness in my heart that can't be healed from medicine. No chemo, drug, or miraculous homeopathic pill can take it away. No narcotic is strong enough to dull the pain.

My patients are the medicine I need. Elderly ladies with blue hair that want to hold my hand and call me "honey" because no one is with them. The old men with salt and pepper sprinkled on the few hairs they have left tell me a joke because their children are too busy to listen. The young people who are having surgery because they were reckless, the ones I caution and catch myself preaching to—these are the patients that fill my void.

I preoped a young man last week. Inside the paisley curtains, he cursed as he shook his head side to side and moaned, sounding more like a pop star singing a song of love and loss.

"Help me, someone, I can't take this pain any longer," he yelled.

I pulled a chair close to his bed, placed a cool wash cloth across his forehead and injected morphine into his vein. I asked him how the accident happened.

"I was riding my dirt bike out in the desert and got carried away performing some fancy stunts. I fractured my left leg."

I looked at the external fixator attached to his leg, the swelling in his ankle and knee, and the metal pins that disappeared in his bone. I watched his temple pulsating and thought about life, about luck, about my son, and wondered why he had to die.

I TOOK HIS CALLOUSED hand in mine and listened as he talked about the accident.

"I don't know what happened, the bike just got away from me," he said.

The connection between my patient and Sky went deeper than motorcycles, their bushy eyebrows, big brown eyes and olive complexion, a build referred to as "buff." I wanted to save this patient from a worse fate. I wanted his parents to be immune to the disease that afflicted me. "You're playing Russian Roulette with your life," I told him. I felt his hand squeeze mine. His forehead dripped with tiny beads of perspiration. "My belief is we all die when our time is up. I'm not afraid of death," he said. "We all have to die sometime."

I wanted to put my arms around him and talk about a son who followed that belief. A son who thought he had nine lives and joked about his luck—a son who had two motorcycle accidents before the fatal one. A son who kissed me on the cheek two days before he died for no particular reason. Instead, I told him to be careful. I don't want to burden others with my grief.

Nine years have passed since Sky's death, but the sense of loss lingers, like a potpourri scent that never quite goes away. I want to be reminded of him, the joys and the heartbreaks. I want to be around others with his interests, language, gestures that link them as one. And just like a child that grows up and leaves, so do the patients with whom I connect. They come and go like the change of seasons—something to count on, like the first rainfall of the year, or the scent of an early bloom leaving us with a bouquet to remember. What remains at the heart of this is its humanity, its search for connections within the seasons of our lives.

Combing Her Hair

~

Mary DeLisle-Berry

I KNOCKED ON THE door and a man answered. He invited me in. His name, he said, was Hank. He was the husband of the patient I was going to meet for the first time that day.

I am an RN and I had been assigned as the case manager for a 56-year-old woman named Maryanne. She had a diagnosis of pancreatic cancer. Hank told me his wife was upstairs and he asked if I would like a cup of coffee before I went up to meet her.

I like to get to know the family early into my relationship with my clients. Hospice is a collaborative venture with patient, family, and the hospice staff. Hospice provides the teaching and the medical supplies needed for end of life care. Nursing, social work, chaplaincy, and volunteer staff offer physical, emotional, and spiritual care and support when they visit. But family and friends are the primary care providers. They are the ones there 24/7 to meet the daily needs of that person and support them through the dying process. They likely will be at bedside when their loved one dies; they will dial the phone and make the call to hospice when that happens.

I sat down, took my coffee with cream, and Hank and I chatted. He was a nice man. Quite a talker. I don't really recall what we talked about. After about 10 minutes or so of small talk, I thanked him for the coffee, got up from the kitchen table, and went up the stairs to meet his wife. I had no idea then what an adventure I had ahead of me. It forever changed my life, deepening my awareness of the power of love.

Maryanne was a matter of fact "don't-bullshit-me" woman. She asked me "How long do I have to live?" shortly after my Avon-lady "Hi my name is Mary. I'm your hospice nurse" intro. Okay, I thought, apparently no time was going to be spent here chit-chatting with Maryanne.

When I mentioned how I enjoyed meeting her husband Hank, she said that I had "talked more with Hank in the last 10 minutes" than she had "in the last 10 years." Interesting, I thought, particularly because

Hank ultimately was going to assume the role of primary caregiver.

I stumbled through that first visit with Maryanne—she was very guarded. No touchy-feely stuff wafting in the air. No hand-holding. She wanted a schedule of when I would be visiting, a list of the meds she would be taking, and to be kept informed about how long she had to live and how she would die; she specifically wanted to know what would happen physiologically that would cause her death. "Don't spare any details," she instructed. So we made a schedule for my visits, we reviewed her medications, and I agreed to be totally honest and straight-forward with the information she wanted from me. She had clearly defined what she wanted from hospice; I was clearly committed to providing hospice care for her—her way. The dance had begun.

EARLY IN MY VISITS with Maryanne, during every visit, she was very insistent that I increase the dose of her Morphine and Ativan. I would bring her request to our hospice doctor, and her pain and anti-anxiety medications were taken up with her request. Pain and anxiety are what the patient says they are, and hospice is about meeting comfort needs and managing pain. But during my visits after these increases in dosage, all I ever observed was my patient getting more and more "dopey."

On one of these visits she slurred out the question, "How long 'til I die?" I'd gotten to know her well enough by then I felt I knew how to answer that one. We had actually established a good rapport and had discussed many of her beliefs about life and death. So I said, "Well, unless you drown from drooling, or pass out and fall into your oatmeal and meet the same fate, I suspect it is going to be awhile yet." That woke her up a bit.

I explained graphically, as I agreed at the beginning I would, that physiologically her body still had body fat to burn and it had the ability to use that fat for energy. Her body was not burning muscle yet. Her heart was a muscle, and it was strong. I was speaking her language. I knew we were connecting. "You are not leaving any time soon as far as I can see," I said. She got teary-eyed.

It wasn't physical pain she was trying to get rid of: It was fear she was trying to medicate away. She said so after my seemingly rude and to the point reply to her question. It was an effective pattern interrupt. And she got it. What she was doing was not working. I then asked her if she would like to explore a few other ways to manage some of this fear. She said yes. And I believe at that point hospice spun its magic, and the dignity and grace Maryanne and her family deserved to experience at her end of life journey began.

Maryanne was a part of the Baha'i faith. Friends from her congregation would come to visit. They brought food and little gifts of inspirational readings to offer support to her. She had been involved for years with the Baha'i faith and was a very active member in their local community. She told me she had always found strength and purpose for her life integrating her faith into her everyday life. But when she was diagnosed with cancer her entire focus had gotten stuck on "when and how will I die?"

She wasn't able to take in the love and comfort from her friends. When they came over she was "drugged." She was unable to quiet her mind long enough to think about anything else. Her actually physical pain was managed very well. Her spiritual pain was raging, but her source for addressing that pain was blocked. None of the drugs she was taking could manage that kind of pain.

Because she had agreed to try some alternative symptom management, I suggested guided imagery. Perhaps she could relax and that might open a pathway for her to quiet her mind and find strength again in the things that had sustained her through out her life. She was very receptive to that idea. She had used hypnosis many years prior to quit smoking and was pleased at how well that had worked for her.

A session of guided imagery was held at her bedside and taped for her; it was scripted by her, for her, specifically using her favorite imaginings: thoughts and ideas that brought her peace of mind and hope were used to help her remember how she had lived her life before fear had taken over.

I remember very well one story she wanted on that tape to help her relax: she said her father was a fisherman. When she was a little girl she would sit on the dock and watch for him to come in with his boat at the end of the day. It was a carefree time in her life when she felt safe and loved. So that is the story we used to promote relaxation on the tape. We put some of her favorite poems and songs and spiritual quotes into the tape as well. It was her tape, done her way.

She loved it! She listened to it when she felt anxious, when she went to sleep at night, when she wanted to catnap during the day. She fell into the experience of relaxing with it. And slowly over the weeks that followed she had us wean her medications down to levels that managed her pain, and yet allowed her to be present and alert for her life. She started enjoying the visits from her friends. She was even talking to Hank. One day when I came to visit, Hank was combing her hair. It made me cry.

Not all of my experiences in hospice have been so dramatic. But they have all been unique. And sacred. Seeing "don't-bullshit-me" Maryanne having her hair brushed by a man she said she had barely spoke to in the past ten years touched me deeply. Later, after her death when I met her two grown daughters, they told me of some very amazing conversations they had with their mom during those months prior to her death. They told me how "stunned" they were observing tenderness between their parents during that time. One daughter said her mom and dad seemed to have "fallen in love again"—something she never thought she would see.

I honestly do not know how all that healing happened between them. I'm guessing Maryanne and Hank must have called a truce at one point to the silence and done some talking with each other. He did become her caregiver. Bathing her, helping to feed her, sitting vigil many hours at her bedside. It was Hank who made the call to hospice when she died.

What I do know is that Maryanne knew what she needed to do to make peace with her life and her death. She was stuck, and hospice brought some ideas in to help her get through the stuckness so she could tap her own wellspring of strength and hope and courage. And she did.

A Call to Nursing
Stories about Challenge and Commitment

~

Paula Sergi, BSN, MFA
Geraldine Gorman, RN, PhD

EDITORS

WHAT LEADS A person to become a nurse? Hear from nurses themselves about why they joined the field and why some of them have decided to leave. Nurses new to the profession and those who have practiced for decades reveal what it is really like to be a nurse. They share true stories of the patients and colleagues who have impacted their careers, as well as the challenges specific to their specialties or the settings in which they work. Startlingly honest, *A Call to Nursing* offers fascinating insights into the lives of nurses.

IN STORES ~ SPRING 2009!

New Lives
Nurses' Stories about Babies

~

Kathleen Huggins, RN, MS
EDITOR

IN THE FIRST 28 days of an infant's life, neonatal nurses, perinatal nurses, midwives, ob-gyns, labor and delivery nurses, pediatric nurses, lactation consultants, nurse practitioners, postpartum nurses, and others in the nursing field play a critical role in helping parents care for these new lives. In this remarkable collection of true stories, nurses share the unique clinical and emotional challenges of caring for infants, and what they have learned along the way.

Share Your Stories
with Kaplan Publishing

KAPLAN PUBLISHING, THE #1 educational resource for nurses, would like to feature your story in an upcoming anthology in the *Kaplan Voices: Nurses* series. Please share the stories behind the relationships, experiences, and issues you encounter on the job—whether you work in a hospital, clinic, home setting, hospice, private medical practice, or elsewhere.

Entertaining and educational, inspirational and practical, each *Kaplan Voices: Nurses* anthology features true stories written by nurses about the experiences and relationships that inspire and enrich their lives and all those who come into contact with them.

FOR WRITER'S GUIDELINES or to join our mailing list, please contact Kaplan Publishing by email at: kaplanvoicesnurses@gmail.com, or write to us at:

Nurse Stories
Editorial Assistant
Kaplan Publishing
1 Liberty Plaza, 24th Floor
New York, NY 10006, USA

More Nursing Books
Available From Kaplan

Notes on Nursing
Florence Nightingale
978-1-4277-9791-1 $9.95

Your Career in Nursing, 5th Edition
Annetee Vallano, MS, RN, CS
978-1-427-9787-2 $17.00

First Year Nurse
Barbara Arnoldussen, RN, MBA
978-1-4195-5116-1 $12.00

How to Survive Clinical
Diann Martin
978-1-4277-9822-0 $12.95

Labor of Love: A Midwife's Memoir
Cara Muhlhahn, CNM
978-1-4277-9821-3 $25.95   (available January 2009)

Saving Lives: Why the Media's Portrayal of Nurses Puts Us All at Risk
Sandy Summers, MSN, MPH, RN
Harry Jacob Summers, JD
978-1-4277-9845-9 $24.95   (available January 2009)

AVAILABLE WHEREVER BOOKS ARE SOLD!